Disclaimer

This book is intended to provide helpful and informative material on the subject of nutrition and health. It is presented with the understanding that the authors and publishers are not engaged in rendering medical, health, psychological, or any other kind of personal professional services in the book. If the reader requires personal medical, health, or other assistance or advice, a competent professional should be consulted.

The authors and publisher specifically disclaim all responsibility for any liability, loss, or risk, personal or otherwise, which is incurred as a consequence, directly or indirectly, of the use and application of any of the contents of this book.

Furthermore, information regarding dietary supplements, health strategies, and nutrition may change, and the reader is advised that this book does not contain all the relevant information concerning the subjects discussed.

Recipes included in this book should be used at the reader's own risk. The ingredients or techniques mentioned might cause allergic reactions or other medical issues. Always consult with a medical professional before making any significant changes to your diet or lifestyle, especially if you have underlying health conditions.

While the authors and publishers have made every effort to ensure the accuracy and completeness of the information contained in this book, we do not guarantee or warrant the accuracy thereof, nor are we responsible for any errors or omissions, or for the results obtained from the use of such information.

By reading and using this book, you agree that neither the authors nor the publisher nor any of their employees, partners, or agents are responsible for the success or failure of your decisions relating to any information presented by this book.

Contents

Preface

Welcome to "Food Swap: Your Guide to Replacing Junk Food with Healthy Choices," a journey into transforming your eating habits one delicious swap at a time. The essence of this book is built on a simple yet profound concept: swapping out less nutritious foods for healthier alternatives. This is not about strict diets or depriving yourself but about making smarter, sustainable changes that enhance your health and well-being.

The idea for this book originated from my personal experiences and challenges with maintaining a balanced diet amidst a busy lifestyle. Like many, I found myself reaching for quick, convenient foods, which often meant processed snacks, fast food, and sugary beverages.

The impact of these choices became evident not just in my physical health but in my energy levels, mood, and overall well-being. The turning point came when my doctor highlighted the stark reality during a routine check-up: continue down this path, and face a future rife with health issues.

Determined to change my course but overwhelmed by the plethora of diet advice, I sought a simpler solution. That's when I discovered the power of food swapping. It started small: whole grain bread instead of white, water instead of soda, fruit instead of candy.

These swaps gradually built up, leading to more significant changes that were both manageable and sustainable. The results were not just visible in my health screenings but in how I felt every day—more energetic, clearer skin, better sleep, and a more positive outlook on life.

This book aims to share the simplicity and effectiveness of food swapping, breaking down the science of why certain foods are less beneficial and providing you with easy alternatives that pack a nutritional punch.

Each chapter is designed to help you understand and implement swaps in every meal—from breakfast cereals laden with sugar to wholesome oatmeal that keeps you full longer, from greasy fast-food lunches to nourishing salads that fuel your afternoons, from sodium-heavy dinners to fresh, vibrant dishes that satisfy without the bloat.

The benefits of making these swaps are backed by solid research. Numerous studies have shown that replacing high-calorie, nutrient-poor foods with nutrient-dense alternatives can lead to better weight management, reduced risk of chronic diseases such as diabetes, heart disease, and certain cancers, and improved mental health. This book delves into these studies, offering you a clear picture of how food influences our bodies and minds.

I've included examples of food labels and all-natural products from Traverse Bay Farms, a nationally award-winning gourmet food brand known for its small-batch excellence. Traverse Bay Farms is committed to sustainability and eco-friendly practices. They prioritize using locally grown produce wherever possible.

If you choose to order from them, they can usually ship your entire order in a single box directly to your door, minimizing environmental impact, supporting American farmers, and allowing you to enjoy their award-winning gourmet food products at every meal. For more information, you can visit their website at www.TraverseBayFarms.com or call them at 1-877-746-7477.

"Food Swap" is more than just a guide; it's a tool to revolutionize your diet. It's designed for real people living real lives. Whether you're a busy professional, a parent juggling the demands of family life, or someone simply looking to feel better in their skin, the swaps here are for you. They are practical, doable, and most importantly, effective.

Join me on this path to healthier eating. It's not about perfection but progress. With each swap, you'll be taking a step towards a healthier you, not just for today but for a lifetime. Let's make these changes together, one swap at a time.

Sincerely,

Mike Oliver

Introduction to the concept of food swapping

Welcome to the transformative world of food swapping, a concept as straightforward as it is effective. At its core, food swapping involves substituting less healthy food choices with healthier alternatives. This simple switch can lead to improved nutrition, better health outcomes, and a more enjoyable eating experience without feeling deprived.

The idea behind food swapping is not about cutting out your favorite foods or adhering to a strict diet that makes you miserable. Instead, it's about making small, manageable changes that collectively have a significant impact on your overall health. It's about choosing whole grain bread over white bread, opting for air-popped popcorn instead of potato chips, or preparing a homemade smoothie rather than grabbing a commercially made milkshake loaded with sugar.

Why does food swapping work? It's grounded in the principle of substitution rather than elimination. When you replace a high-calorie, nutrient-poor item with a nutrient-dense alternative, you reduce the consumption of unhealthy fats, excess sugars, and empty calories.

Simultaneously, you increase your intake of essential nutrients like fiber, vitamins, and minerals without drastically altering your diet. This makes the change sustainable over the long term, rather than a temporary fix that fades once a strict diet is over.

Consider breakfast, often dubbed the most important meal of the day. A common morning rush might have you grabbing a pastry or a sugary cereal. These options are convenient but often lead to a mid-morning energy crash.

Swapping these out for oatmeal topped with fresh berries and a sprinkle of nuts not only sustains your energy levels longer but also contributes to your daily nutritional goals.

Implementing food swaps doesn't just benefit your physical health; it also enhances your mental well-being. Eating a balanced diet with ample nutrients can improve mood and energy levels, making you feel more active and less sluggish. The psychological boost from knowing you're making healthier choices can also be incredibly empowering.

Food swapping is a journey of discovery. It's about exploring new flavors and ingredients, and finding joy in the kitchen again. As we progress through this book, we'll delve deeper into how you can apply this concept to every meal of the day, with practical tips and delicious recipes to guide you.

Let's embark on this path together, transforming our plates to nourish our bodies and enrich our lives.

The motivation behind the book

This book is much more than a compilation of healthy recipes and food swaps; it's rooted in a personal journey—one that transformed not just my diet but my entire approach to living well.

Several years ago, my life was markedly different. Long hours at work were often coupled with even longer periods sitting in traffic, leading me to rely heavily on the convenience of fast food and ready-made meals. Breakfast was often a high-sugar coffee drink; lunch was a grab-and-go affair from whatever was nearby; dinners were late and consisted of whatever I could quickly microwave. I felt constantly tired, my weight was creeping up, and my health markers were headed in the wrong direction.

The wake-up call came during a routine check-up. My doctor was forthright: I was on a fast track to serious health issues if I didn't make changes. But the idea of overhauling my diet was daunting. I wasn't a cook; I had no time, and frankly, I liked the taste of my regular meals. That's when my doctor suggested something that didn't feel so overwhelming: food swapping.

I started small. I swapped my morning pastry for Greek yogurt with fruit and a drizzle of honey. Instead of a fast-food burger at lunch, I began packing whole grain wraps filled with veggies and lean proteins. These small changes were surprisingly doable and even more surprisingly, enjoyable.

The more swaps I made, the better I felt. My energy levels improved, I started losing weight, and my blood work showed significant improvements. These swaps became my new norm, and the benefits were too good to ignore.

Inspired by my own transformation, I wanted to share this approach with others who might be feeling just as overwhelmed as I did. This book aims to demystify healthy eating and show that it can be simple, satisfying, and most importantly, sustainable.

Through "Food Swap," we aspire to pass on the lessons of my journey. Each swap you make brings you a step closer to better health and a more vibrant life. This isn't just my story—it's a path that we can all walk together, one swap at a time.

The health benefits of making smarter food choices

Making smarter food choices is not just about losing weight or fitting into a smaller size; it's about enhancing your overall quality of life. This chapter explores the myriad health benefits that come from replacing junk food with nutritious alternatives. Whether it's improving physical health, boosting mental well-being, or enhancing emotional stability, the impacts are profound and far-reaching.

1. Enhanced Physical Health

Swapping out high-calorie, nutrient-poor foods for healthier alternatives can lead to significant improvements in physical health. One of the most immediate benefits is better weight management. Foods that are high in fiber and protein, such as fruits, vegetables, whole grains, and lean proteins, help you feel fuller longer, reducing the urge to snack on unhealthy options. This can naturally lead to a calorie deficit and subsequent weight loss without the need for restrictive dieting.

Moreover, these healthier food choices contribute to improved heart health. Replacing saturated fats found in fried and processed foods with healthier fats, like those from avocados, nuts, and fish, can lower cholesterol levels and reduce the risk of heart disease. Additionally, a diet rich in fruits, vegetables, and whole grains can improve blood pressure and decrease the risk of developing type 2 diabetes.

2. Mental and Cognitive Benefits

Diet impacts not only the body but also the mind. Foods rich in omega-3 fatty acids, antioxidants, and vitamins have been shown to enhance cognitive function and may even reduce the risk of dementia. Regular consumption of nutrient-dense foods can also stabilize blood sugar, which is crucial for maintaining consistent energy levels and mood.

3. Emotional Well-being

The psychological benefits of making healthier food choices are often overlooked. Diet plays a crucial role in mood regulation and can influence symptoms of depression and anxiety. Foods high in vitamins, minerals, and antioxidants can boost serotonin levels, a neurotransmitter responsible for feelings of well-being and happiness.

4. Long-Term Health Benefits

Finally, committing to smarter food choices has long-term health benefits. It can increase life expectancy, reduce the risk of chronic diseases, improve quality of life in later years, and promote a more active and fulfilling lifestyle.

In summary, the act of swapping junk food for healthy alternatives offers extensive benefits that permeate all aspects of health. It's about making mindful choices that not only nourish your body but also enrich your mind and soothe your soul. This holistic approach to eating can transform not just your physical appearance but also your overall life experience.

Chapter 1: Understanding Nutrition Basics

The Foundations of Nutrition - Macronutrients and Micronutrients

Understanding the role of macronutrients and micronutrients is essential for making informed dietary decisions that support your health and well-being. This chapter dives into the functions, sources, and health impacts of these crucial dietary components.

Macronutrients: The Big Three

1. Carbohydrates

Carbohydrates are the primary energy source for the body. They are broken down into glucose, which fuels our cells, tissues, and organs. Carbohydrates can be classified into two types: simple and complex. Simple carbohydrates, or sugars, are found in foods like fruits, milk, and also refined sugars used in baking and sweets. Complex carbohydrates, or starches, are found in whole grains, legumes, and starchy vegetables like potatoes.

It's essential to prioritize complex carbohydrates because they contain fiber, which helps regulate blood sugar levels and promotes a healthy digestive system. The Dietary Guidelines for Americans recommend that carbohydrates make up about 45% to 65% of your total daily calories (U.S. Department of Health and Human Services, 2020).

2. Proteins

Proteins are the building blocks of the body, crucial for building and repairing tissues, making enzymes and hormones, and supporting immune function. Dietary protein is composed of amino acids, some of which are essential because the body cannot produce them. These must be obtained from food. Good sources of protein include meat, fish, dairy, legumes, and for those following plant-based diets, quinoa and soy products.

The Recommended Dietary Allowance for protein for the average adult is about 0.8 grams per kilogram of body weight per day (Institute of Medicine, Food and Nutrition Board, 2002).

3. Fats

Fats are vital for maintaining energy, supporting cell growth, protecting organs, and keeping the body warm. Fats also help in the absorption of fat-soluble vitamins (A, D, E, K). Dietary fats can be saturated, unsaturated, and trans fats. Unsaturated fats, found in olive oil, avocado, and fish, are beneficial for heart health, while saturated fats should be consumed in moderation, and trans fats avoided.

The American Heart Association recommends that 20% to 35% of your total daily calories should come from fats, primarily the healthier unsaturated types (American Heart Association, 2020).

Micronutrients: Vitamins and Minerals

Vitamins

Vitamins are organic compounds that are crucial for normal cell function, growth, and development. There are 13 essential vitamins, including vitamins A, C, D, E, and K, along with the B vitamins such as riboflavin and folate. Each vitamin has specific roles, such as Vitamin D's importance in bone health and Vitamin C's role in immune function and skin health. A diet rich in fruits, vegetables, lean proteins, and whole grains typically provides adequate amounts of vitamins.

Minerals

Minerals, like vitamins, support the body's processes. Calcium and phosphorus are critical for bone health, iron is needed for blood oxygenation, and zinc supports immune health and wound healing. Minerals are categorized into macrominerals and trace minerals, depending on the amount required by the body. Foods like dairy, fish, and leafy greens are rich in various essential minerals.

Both macronutrients and micronutrients are crucial for maintaining health. While macronutrients provide the necessary energy to function, micronutrients support the body at a cellular level, promoting the repair and maintenance of vital systems. A balanced diet, rich in vegetables, fruits, whole grains, healthy fats, and lean proteins, can typically provide all these nutrients in adequate amounts. Regular dietary adjustments based on lifestyle, health conditions, and age are essential for optimal health.

References:

- U.S. Department of Health and Human Services. (2020). Dietary Guidelines for Americans.
- Institute of Medicine, Food and Nutrition Board. (2002). Dietary Reference Intakes for Energy, Carbohydrate, Fiber, Fat, Fatty Acids, Cholesterol, Protein, and Amino Acids.
- American Heart Association. (2020). Dietary Recommendations for Healthy Children.

The Essential Trio: Fiber, Water, and Antioxidants

A well-balanced diet is not only about what we reduce but also what we must adequately consume. Among the crucial components of a healthy diet are fiber, water, and antioxidants—each playing a unique and vital role in maintaining health and preventing disease. This chapter delves into the importance of these three dietary elements, their benefits, and how to ensure adequate intake.

Fiber: The Unsung Hero of Digestive Health

Dietary fiber refers to plant-based carbohydrates that, unlike other carbs, cannot be digested by your body. Instead, fiber passes relatively intact through your stomach, small intestine, and colon and out of your body.

Fiber is broadly classified into two types: soluble, which dissolves in water, and insoluble, which does not. Soluble fiber helps to soften stool so it can slide through the GI tract more easily, whereas insoluble fiber adds bulk to the stool, helping it pass more quickly and easily.

The benefits of dietary fiber extend beyond simple digestion. Studies have shown that high fiber intakes are associated with significantly lower risks of developing coronary heart disease, stroke, hypertension, diabetes, obesity, and certain gastrointestinal diseases (Anderson et al., 2009).

High fiber foods are also more filling, which helps control appetite and might contribute to weight management. The American Dietetic Association recommends a daily fiber intake of 25 grams for women and 38 grams for men (American Dietetic Association, 2008).

Water: More Than Just Thirst Quencher

Water is crucial for life. It serves many essential functions in your body, including maintaining the health and integrity of every cell, aiding in digestion and the absorption of nutrients, and flushing toxins from the body. Moreover, water helps to regulate body temperature through sweating, lubricates and cushions joints, and supports the body's all-around vital functions (Popkin, D'Anci, and Rosenberg, 2010).

Despite its crucial role, many people do not consume enough water. The National Academies of Sciences, Engineering, and Medicine recommend a daily water intake of about 3.7 liters (or 13 cups) for men and 2.7 liters (or 9 cups) for women from all beverages and foods (National Academies of Sciences, Engineering, and Medicine, 2004).

Antioxidants: The Defense Agents

Antioxidants are compounds that inhibit oxidation, a chemical reaction that can produce free radicals, thereby leading to chain reactions that may damage the cells of organisms. Vitamins A, C, E, and the mineral selenium are among substances that are capable of acting as antioxidants. They play a role in neutralizing free radicals, thus preventing cell damage.

The health benefits of antioxidants are vast; they are believed to help fend off heart disease and cancer, maintain vision, slow down the processes that age us, and more (Pham-Huy et al., 2008). Foods rich in antioxidants include berries, nuts, dark chocolate, spinach, and artichokes. Regular consumption of these foods can contribute significantly to reducing inflammation and protecting the body against various chronic diseases.

In summary, fiber, water, and antioxidants are foundational to good health. Adequate intake of these can help maintain a healthy digestive system, ensure proper hydration, and protect against cellular damage and chronic diseases. By integrating high-fiber foods, adequate water, and antioxidant-rich foods into your diet, you can significantly impact your overall health and well-being.

References:

- Anderson, J.W., Baird, P., Davis, R.H. Jr., Ferreri, S., Knudtson, M., Koraym, A., Waters, V., Williams, C.L. (2009). Health benefits of dietary fiber. *Nutrition Reviews, 67*(4), 188-205.
- American Dietetic Association (2008). Position of the American Dietetic Association: Health Implications of Dietary Fiber.
- Popkin, B.M., D'Anci, K.E., Rosenberg, I.H. (2010). Water, Hydration and Health. *Nutrition Reviews, 68*(8), 439-458.
- National Academies of Sciences, Engineering, and Medicine (2004). Dietary Reference Intakes for Water, Potassium, Sodium, Chloride, and Sulfate.
- Pham-Huy, L.A., He, H., Pham-Huy, C. (2008). Free radicals, antioxidants in disease and health. *International Journal of Biomedical Science, 4*(2), 89-96.

Impact of Food Choices on Health

The impact of dietary choices extends far beyond the immediate pleasure of taste. Our food selections influence various aspects of health, including weight management, energy levels, and the risk of developing chronic diseases. Understanding these relationships can empower us to make choices that enhance our well-being.

Weight Management

Obesity and being overweight are significant risk factors for numerous health issues, including cardiovascular diseases, diabetes, and joint problems. The energy balance equation—calories in versus calories out—dictates weight control, but the quality of calories consumed can influence this balance.

Foods high in refined sugars and fats can lead to weight gain as they are more calorie-dense and less satisfying than whole grains, fruits, and vegetables, which are lower in calories and higher in fiber (Rolls, Ello-Martin, & Tohill, 2004). Therefore, making intelligent food swaps from high-calorie junk foods to nutrient-dense options can aid in maintaining a healthy weight.

Energy Levels

Diet plays a crucial role in energy levels. Foods high in complex carbohydrates, such as whole grains, provide a steady release of glucose into the bloodstream, ensuring a consistent energy supply. In contrast, high-sugar foods cause spikes in blood sugar levels followed by rapid declines, which can lead to fluctuations in energy levels throughout the day (Ludwig, 2002).

Additionally, iron-rich foods like lean meats and spinach are crucial for preventing anemia, a common energy-drainer. Maintaining balanced meals that include a good mix of macronutrients (carbohydrates, proteins, and fats) and micronutrients helps stabilize energy levels and optimize overall vitality.

Chronic Disease Risk

Diet is directly linked to several chronic diseases. For instance, high intakes of saturated fats and trans fats are associated with increased risk of heart disease. Conversely, diets rich in fruits, vegetables, and fatty fishes (which are high in omega-3 fatty acids) can reduce inflammation and decrease the risk of cardiovascular conditions (Hu, Manson, & Willett, 2001).

Similarly, type 2 diabetes can be influenced by diet. Frequent consumption of high-glycemic foods (e.g., white bread, sugary drinks) can lead to higher long-term blood sugar levels, which may increase diabetes risk (Salmerón et al., 1997). By choosing lower-glycemic-index foods and monitoring carbohydrate intake, individuals can manage or even prevent this disease.

Moreover, dietary choices impact cancer risk. Diets high in fruits and vegetables are associated with a lower risk of several types of cancer, likely due to the protective effects of dietary fiber and antioxidants (Block et al., 1992). These substances help to neutralize potentially damaging free radicals in the body, reducing oxidative stress and inflammation, which are linked to cancer progression.

Conclusion

The science is clear: making informed food choices has significant impacts on weight management, energy levels, and chronic disease risk. By understanding the nutritional value of foods and how they affect our bodies, we can make better decisions that contribute to long-term health and vitality. Adopting a diet that emphasizes whole foods over processed ones can lead to a healthier, more vibrant life.

References:

- Rolls, B.J., Ello-Martin, J.A., & Tohill, B.C. (2004). What can intervention studies tell us about the relationship between fruit and vegetable consumption and weight management? *Nutrition Reviews, 62*(1), 1-17.
- Ludwig, D.S. (2002). The glycemic index: physiological mechanisms relating to obesity, diabetes, and cardiovascular disease. *JAMA, 287*(18), 2414-2423.
- Hu, F.B., Manson, J.E., & Willett, W.C. (2001). Types of dietary fat and risk of coronary heart disease: a critical review. *Journal of the American College of Nutrition, 20*(1), 5-19.
- Salmerón, J., Manson, J.E., Stampfer, M.J., Colditz, G.A., Wing, A.L., & Willett, W.C. (1997). Dietary fiber, glycemic load, and risk of non-insulin-dependent diabetes mellitus in women. *JAMA, 277*(6), 472-477.
- Block, G., Patterson, B., & Subar, A. (1992). Fruit, vegetables, and cancer prevention: a review of the epidemiological evidence. *Nutrition and Cancer, 18*(1), 1-29.

Chapter 2: The Art of Food Swapping

Principles of successful food swaps

Incorporating healthier food choices into your diet does not need to be a daunting task. Successful food swapping is about making smart substitutions that can enhance your nutritional intake without sacrificing flavor or satisfaction. This chapter outlines the key principles of successful food swaps, complete with practical checklists to guide you in making these changes effortlessly.

1. Prioritize Nutrient Density

Principle: Choose foods that offer more nutrients per calorie. Nutrient-dense foods provide vitamins, minerals, fiber, and other beneficial substances with relatively few calories.

To-Do List:

- Swap white rice for quinoa or brown rice to increase your fiber and protein intake.
- Replace regular pasta with whole wheat pasta or spiralized vegetables like zucchini for a lower calorie, higher fiber alternative.
- Opt for lean meats such as chicken or turkey breast instead of higher-fat cuts or processed meats.

2. Understand Portion Sizes

Principle: Managing portion sizes is crucial, even when making healthier choices, to avoid consuming excess calories.

Checklist:

- Use smaller plates to help control portion sizes naturally.
- Measure out servings of snacks like nuts or seeds to avoid overeating.
- Familiarize yourself with the serving sizes on nutrition labels and adjust your portions accordingly.

3. Reduce Added Sugars

Principle: Decreasing intake of added sugars can significantly benefit your overall health, reducing risks for diabetes, obesity, and heart disease (Johnson et al., 2009).

To-Do List:

- Substitute sugary cereals with oatmeal flavored with fresh fruit or a small amount of honey.
- Choose plain yogurt instead of flavored yogurts packed with sugar; sweeten it naturally with fruit or a drizzle of maple syrup.
- Swap soda or fruit juice for water, unsweetened iced tea, or infused water.

4. Favor Whole Foods Over Processed

Principle: Whole foods are closer to their natural state and tend not to contain the added salts, sugars, and fats found in processed foods, which can be detrimental to health (Monteiro et al., 2018).

Checklist:

- Opt for fresh or frozen fruits and vegetables instead of canned versions that may contain added sugars or sodium.
- Select whole grains rather than refined grains to maximize nutritional content.
- Prepare homemade meals whenever possible to control the quality and quantity of ingredients.

5. Incorporate Healthy Fats

Principle: Not all fats are created equal. Healthy fats, such as those found in avocados, nuts, seeds, and fatty fish, play a vital role in heart health and overall well-being (Mozaffarian & Wu, 2011).

To-Do List:

- Use avocado or hummus as a spread instead of butter or margarine.
- Include a portion of fatty fish like salmon or mackerel in your meals twice a week.
- Cook with olive oil instead of butter or other saturated fats.

6. Stay Flexible and Creative

Principle: Making food swaps should not feel restrictive but rather like a creative and enjoyable endeavor.

Checklist:

- Experiment with herbs and spices to flavor dishes instead of relying on salt or sugar.
- Try new fruits and vegetables regularly to keep meals interesting and varied.
- If a swap doesn't work for you, be flexible and try different options until you find what satisfies your taste and nutritional needs.

Conclusion

Adopting these principles requires thoughtful choices and sometimes a bit of creativity, but the health benefits are well worth the effort. By making these swaps part of your routine, you'll find that eating healthily can also be delicious and satisfying.

References:

- Johnson, R.K., Appel, L.J., Brands, M., Howard, B.V., Lefevre, M., Lustig, R.H., Sacks, F., Steffen, L.M., & Wylie-Rosett, J. (2009). Dietary sugars intake and cardiovascular health: A scientific statement from the American Heart Association. *Circulation, 120*(11), 1011-1020.
- Monteiro, C.A., Cannon, G., Levy, R.B., Moubarac, J.C., Jaime, P., Martins, A.P., Canella, D., Louzada, M., & Parra, D. (2018). Ultra-processed foods: What they are and how to identify them. *Public Health Nutrition, 22*(5), 936-941.
- Mozaffarian, D., & Wu, J.H.Y. (2011). Omega-3 fatty acids and cardiovascular disease: Effects on risk factors, molecular pathways, and clinical events. *Journal of the American College of Cardiology, 58*(20), 2047-2067.

Decoding food labels - Identifying less healthy options

Understanding food labels is a critical skill for making informed dietary choices. Food labels provide essential information about the nutritional content of a product, helping you to avoid less healthy options laden with excess fats, sugars, and sodium. This chapter guides you through the key components of food labels and how to interpret them effectively.

1. Serving Size and Servings Per Container

Principle: Always start by looking at the serving size and the number of servings per container. These figures are crucial because all the nutritional information provided on the label is based on one serving of the food.

Checklist:

- Compare the serving size on the label to the amount you actually eat. If you typically eat double the serving size listed, you need to double the nutritional values to get an accurate picture of what you're consuming.
- Be particularly cautious with items that appear to be single servings but contain multiple servings per package.

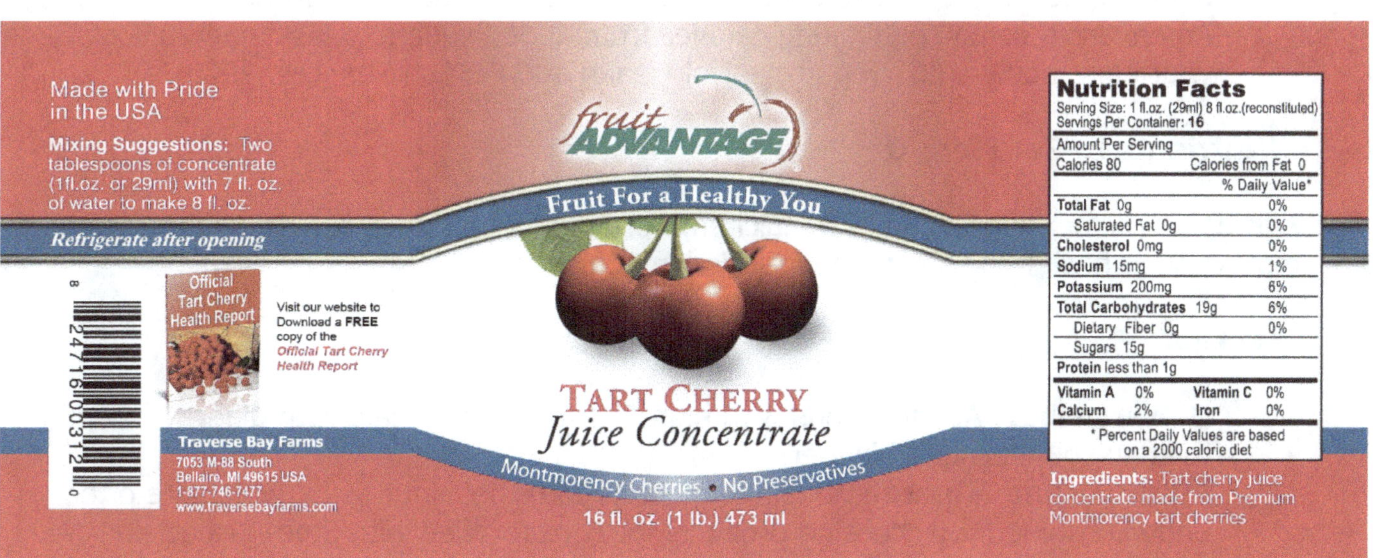

2. Calories

Principle: Calories provide a measure of how much energy you get from a serving of this food. Knowing the calorie content can help you manage your energy intake, which is crucial for maintaining healthy body weight.

Checklist:

- Identify how many calories are in one serving.
- Determine if the calorie amount is appropriate for your dietary needs, considering your total daily calorie goal.

3. Nutrients to Limit

Principle: Certain nutrients, including fats, sodium, and sugars, should be limited as part of a healthy diet. High intake of these can lead to weight gain, heart disease, high blood pressure, and other health issues (U.S. FDA, 2018).

Checklist:

- **Total Fat**: Look for foods with lower amounts of saturated and trans fats. Choose products with higher unsaturated fats.
- **Sodium**: Seek options with 140 mg of sodium per serving or less, as these are considered low sodium.
- **Sugars**: Be wary of added sugars. The 2020-2025 Dietary Guidelines for Americans recommend limiting calories from added sugars to less than 10% of your daily intake (U.S. Department of Health and Human Services, 2020).

4. Nutrients to Get More Of

Principle: Dietary fiber, vitamin D, calcium, iron, and potassium are nutrients that can improve your health and should be included in your diet.

Checklist:

- **Dietary Fiber**: Aim for foods with high fiber content to help with digestion and to keep you feeling full longer.
- **Vitamins and Minerals**: Ensure you're getting these nutrients, which are often underconsumed, by choosing products that are fortified with them, especially vitamin D and calcium.

5. Ingredients List

Principle: The ingredients list on a food label tells you everything that is in the food, by weight, from highest to lowest. This list can reveal added sugars, unhealthy fats, and artificial ingredients that might not be obvious from the nutrient list.

Checklist:

- Look for whole foods as the first ingredients, such as whole grains, meats, or whole fruits and vegetables.
- Avoid products with long lists of additives, artificial flavors, or preservatives.
- Be alert for different names for sugar, such as high fructose corn syrup, agave nectar, or cane juice.

Conclusion

By understanding how to read and interpret food labels, you can make healthier choices that align with your nutritional goals. This knowledge enables you to identify and limit the intake of less healthy food options, thereby enhancing your overall diet quality.

References:

- U.S. Food and Drug Administration (FDA). (2018). How to Understand and Use the Nutrition Facts Label.
- U.S. Department of Health and Human Services. (2020). Dietary Guidelines for Americans 2020-2025.

Balancing taste, convenience, and nutrition

Creating a diet that is delicious, convenient, and nutritious is one of the key challenges in adopting healthier eating habits. However, it is possible to find a balance that satisfies the palate, fits into a busy lifestyle, and delivers the nutrients your body needs. This chapter explores strategies for achieving this balance, enhancing both the enjoyment and healthfulness of your meals.

1. Emphasizing Flavor Through Healthy Ingredients

Principle: The misconception that healthy food cannot be tasty stems from unfamiliarity with the right ingredients and cooking methods. Using herbs, spices, and seasonings can enhance the natural flavors of food without adding excessive calories or sodium.

Checklist:

- Experiment with a variety of herbs and spices like basil, cinnamon, cumin, and chili powder to find combinations that you enjoy.
- Use techniques like roasting or grilling to enhance the natural sweetness and flavors of vegetables and meats.
- Incorporate umami-rich ingredients such as tomatoes, mushrooms, and low-sodium soy sauce to deepen flavors without relying on salt.

References:

- Drewnowski, A., & Fulgoni, V. (2014). Nutrient profiling of foods: creating a nutrient-rich food index. *Nutrition Reviews, 72*(1), 23-38.

2. Planning for Convenience

Principle: The key to maintaining a healthy diet despite a hectic schedule is preparation. Meal prepping and planning can make nutritious foods as convenient as grabbing a fast-food meal.

Checklist:

- Dedicate time each week to plan meals and prepare ingredients ahead of time.
- Cook in bulk and use portion control to create grab-and-go meals for the week.
- Keep healthy snacks like cut vegetables, nuts, and fruit on hand to avoid reaching for less healthy options.

References:

- American Heart Association. (2021). Meal Planning for Real Life: Tips for Your Budget & Busy Schedule.

3. Ensuring Nutritional Adequacy

Principle: A balanced diet should provide all the necessary nutrients to support bodily functions. This includes macronutrients (proteins, fats, carbohydrates) and micronutrients (vitamins, minerals).

Checklist:

- Include a variety of food groups in each meal to cover a broader spectrum of nutrients.
- Opt for whole grains, lean proteins, healthy fats, and a colorful array of fruits and vegetables.
- Use fortified foods or supplements if necessary to meet the recommended daily intake of key nutrients like vitamin D and omega-3 fatty acids.

References:

- Institute of Medicine. (2005). Dietary Reference Intakes for Energy, Carbohydrate, Fiber, Fat, Fatty Acids, Cholesterol, Protein, and Amino Acids (Macronutrients).

4. Integrating Dietary Preferences and Restrictions

Principle: Tailoring your diet to include personal preferences and dietary restrictions can help sustain long-term adherence and enjoyment.

Checklist:

- Identify personal likes and dislikes, as well as any dietary restrictions (e.g., allergies, lactose intolerance) and find healthy options that cater to these needs.
- Consider cultural preferences and seasonal availability of foods to enhance variety and enjoyment.
- Engage with community resources or online platforms for recipe ideas that cater to specific dietary needs.

References:

- Fanzo, J. (2020). Can diets be healthy, sustainable, and equitable? *Current Obesity Reports, 9*, 495-503.

Conclusion

Balancing taste, convenience, and nutrition is essential for creating a sustainable and enjoyable eating pattern. By strategically utilizing flavorful ingredients, planning ahead, ensuring nutritional adequacy, and catering to personal preferences, you can develop a diet that enhances your health without compromising on taste or convenience.

Chapter 3: Breakfast - Start Your Day Right

Common unhealthy breakfast foods and their pitfalls

Breakfast is often hailed as the most important meal of the day, setting the tone for energy levels and dietary habits. However, many common breakfast foods are far from the healthy start that our bodies need.

This chapter delves into the unhealthy breakfast options that are popular in many diets, discussing their nutritional pitfalls and the impact they can have on health.

1. Sugary Cereals

Pitfall: Many cereals, especially those marketed towards children, contain high levels of added sugars and minimal fiber. Consuming such cereals can lead to spikes in blood sugar and insulin, which can increase the risk of insulin resistance, obesity, and type 2 diabetes over time (Malik et al., 2010).

Healthier Swap: Opt for whole-grain cereals with no added sugars. Enhance flavor with fresh fruits and a sprinkle of cinnamon rather than relying on pre-sweetened options.

References:

- Malik, V. S., Popkin, B. M., Bray, G. A., Després, J. P., Willett, W. C., & Hu, F. B. (2010). Sugar-sweetened beverages, obesity, type 2 diabetes mellitus, and cardiovascular disease risk. *Circulation, 121*(11), 1356-1364.

2. Processed Breakfast Meats

Pitfall: Processed meats like bacon and sausages are high in sodium and saturated fats, and they often contain chemicals like nitrates and nitrites, which have been linked to an increased risk of cancers, particularly colorectal cancer (Micha et al., 2010).

Healthier Swap: Choose lean proteins like turkey bacon or plant-based sausages that offer the satisfaction of meat without the harmful additives and high levels of saturated fats.

References:

- Micha, R., Wallace, S. K., & Mozaffarian, D. (2010). Red and processed meat consumption and risk of incident coronary heart disease, stroke, and diabetes mellitus: a systematic review and meta-analysis. *Circulation, 121*(21), 2271-2283.

3. High-Sugar Granola Bars

Pitfall: Despite their reputation as a healthy snack or breakfast option, many granola bars are loaded with added sugars and unhealthy fats. These can contribute to weight gain and provide little in terms of sustained energy or nutritional value.

Healthier Swap: Make your own granola bars with oats, nuts, seeds, and natural sweeteners like honey to control the amount of sugar and improve the nutritional content.

4. Store-Bought Breakfast Pastries

Pitfall: Muffins, doughnuts, and pastries commonly found at coffee shops are typically made with refined flours, trans fats, and a large amount of sugar. These ingredients contribute to poor heart health, weight gain, and spikes in blood sugar (St-Onge et al., 2007).

Healthier Swap: Bake your own pastries using whole wheat flour, natural sweeteners, and healthy fats like avocado or applesauce to replace butter.

References:

- St-Onge, M. P., Keller, K. L., & Heymsfield, S. B. (2007). Changes in childhood food consumption patterns: a cause for concern in light of increasing body weights. *American Journal of Clinical Nutrition, 86*(6), 1708-1716.

5. Flavored Non-Dairy Creamers

Pitfall: Non-dairy creamers can contain a cocktail of unhealthy ingredients, including trans fats, added sugars, and artificial additives, which can affect cholesterol levels and increase the risk of heart disease.

Healthier Swap: Use natural alternatives like almond milk, oat milk, or a small amount of real cream. Sweeten your coffee with a dash of cinnamon or vanilla extract for flavor without the health risks.

Conclusion

Understanding the nutritional pitfalls of common breakfast choices is crucial for making better decisions that align with health goals. By recognizing these unhealthy options and implementing the suggested healthier swaps, individuals can enjoy a nutritious breakfast that supports their overall well-being. This proactive approach to breakfast can help set a positive tone for nutritious eating throughout the day.

Healthy swap options for breakfast favorites

A nutritious breakfast sets the stage for a day filled with healthy choices. Many traditional breakfast foods, however, are laden with sugars, unhealthy fats, and refined grains. This chapter provides practical swap options for popular breakfast items like cereals, pancakes, and pastries, enabling you to start your day with a meal that is as wholesome as it is delicious.

1. Cereals

Traditional Choice: Many commercial cereals are high in added sugars and low in fiber and protein, which can lead to a spike and then a drop in blood sugar levels, resulting in mid-morning energy crashes.

Healthy Swap:

- **Choose cereals with a whole grain as the first ingredient** and with less than 5 grams of sugar per serving. Brands like Ezekiel 4:9 and Barbara's Puffins offer nutritious options.
- **Enhance flavor naturally by adding fresh fruits**, nuts, or a sprinkle of cinnamon.

2. Pancakes

Traditional Choice: Standard pancakes often rely on refined flour and are typically served with syrup, contributing to high intake of processed carbs and sugars.

Healthy Swap:

- **Use whole grain, oatmeal, or almond flour** to increase fiber and nutrient content.
- **Top pancakes with fresh berries, a dollop of Greek yogurt, or a drizzle of pure maple syrup** instead of the artificially flavored varieties.

3. Pastries

Traditional Choice: Pastries like doughnuts and croissants are high in sugar and trans fats, making them a less than ideal option for a healthy start to the day.

Healthy Swap:

- **Bake your own pastries using whole wheat** or almond flour, and swap out sugar with alternatives like apple sauce or ripe bananas.
- **Use heart-healthy fats** like avocado oil or coconut oil in your baking.
- **Create fillings from fresh fruits** or make your own low-sugar jams.

4. Muffins

Traditional Choice: Store-bought muffins often contain as much sugar as a dessert.

Healthy Swap:

- **Prepare homemade muffins using oat flour or whole wheat flour** which are better for blood sugar control.
- **Incorporate nutrient-dense ingredients** like blueberries, bananas, and zucchini.
- **Sweeten with natural sweeteners** like honey or pure maple syrup in moderation.

5. Bagels

Traditional Choice: Bagels are typically made from refined wheat and are dense in calories, contributing significantly to daily carbohydrate intake.

Healthy Swap:

- **Opt for whole-grain bagels** or those made from alternative flours like spelt.
- **Top with nutrient-rich toppings** such as avocado, smoked salmon, or a light spread of cream cheese and cucumber.

Checklist for Implementing Healthy Breakfast Swaps:

- Read labels carefully — opt for items with whole foods as the top ingredients and without added sugars.
- Increase fiber intake by choosing whole grains over refined grains.
- Enhance flavors with natural options (e.g., fruits, nuts, spices) instead of processed additives or high-sugar toppings.
- Prepare batches of healthier versions of your favorites, like pancakes or muffins, on weekends for easy breakfasts throughout the week.
- Keep a variety of fruits and vegetables on hand to incorporate into breakfast meals, increasing vitamin and mineral intake.

By adopting these healthy swaps, you not only enjoy a delicious breakfast but also contribute positively to your overall health and energy levels throughout the day. Embracing these changes can lead to improved nutrient intake and better eating habits, setting a healthy tone for the day ahead.

Recipes and ideas for quick and nutritious breakfasts

Here are five nutritious and healthy breakfast recipes, each crafted with just five ingredients to keep things simple yet delicious. These recipes are designed to provide a balanced start to your day with minimal fuss.

1. Greek Yogurt Parfait

Ingredients:

- 1 cup Greek yogurt (plain, unsweetened)
- ½ cup mixed berries (strawberries, blueberries, raspberries)
- ¼ cup granola
- 1 tablespoon honey
- 1 tablespoon chia seeds

Instructions:

1. Layer the Greek yogurt at the bottom of a glass or bowl.
2. Add a layer of mixed berries over the yogurt.
3. Sprinkle granola evenly over the berries.
4. Drizzle honey on top for a touch of sweetness.
5. Finish with a sprinkle of chia seeds for added fiber and omega-3s.

2. Avocado Toast with Egg

Ingredients:

- 1 slice whole grain bread
- ½ ripe avocado
- 1 large egg, cooked to your preference (fried, poached, or scrambled)
- Salt and pepper, to taste
- Red pepper flakes (optional, for garnish)

Instructions:

1. Toast the bread to your liking.
2. Mash the avocado and spread it evenly over the toast.
3. Top with the cooked egg.
4. Season with salt, pepper, and red pepper flakes for a bit of spice.

3. Banana Oatmeal Pancakes

Ingredients:

- 1 large ripe banana, mashed
- 2 eggs
- ½ cup rolled oats
- 1 teaspoon vanilla extract
- ¼ teaspoon cinnamon

Instructions:

1. In a bowl, combine the mashed banana, eggs, rolled oats, vanilla extract, and cinnamon.
2. Heat a non-stick skillet over medium heat and spoon the batter to form pancakes.
3. Cook for about 2-3 minutes on each side or until pancakes are golden brown.
4. Serve warm with a drizzle of maple syrup or honey if desired.

4. Smoothie Bowl

Ingredients:

- 1 cup frozen mixed berries
- 1 ripe banana
- ½ cup unsweetened almond milk
- 1 tablespoon almond butter
- 1 tablespoon flaxseed meal

Instructions:

1. Blend the frozen berries, banana, almond milk, and almond butter until smooth.
2. Pour the smoothie into a bowl.
3. Sprinkle flaxseed meal on top.
4. Add additional toppings like nuts, seeds, or more fresh fruit if desired.

5. Cottage Cheese with Pineapple

Ingredients:

- 1 cup low-fat cottage cheese
- ½ cup chopped fresh pineapple
- 1 tablespoon honey or maple syrup
- 1 teaspoon chia seeds
- 1 tablespoon shredded coconut

Instructions:

1. Place the cottage cheese in a serving bowl.
2. Top with chopped pineapple.
3. Drizzle honey or maple syrup over the pineapple and cottage cheese.
4. Sprinkle with chia seeds and shredded coconut for texture and extra flavor.

Each of these breakfast recipes is easy to prepare, providing a healthy mix of proteins, fats, and carbohydrates to start the day energized and satisfied.

Chapter 4: Lunch - Fuel Your Afternoon

Overcoming challenges of eating a healthy lunch on-the-go or at work

Eating a nutritious lunch during a busy workday can be a significant challenge. Many of us find ourselves grabbing the quickest, and often unhealthiest, options available due to time constraints and limited choices. This chapter explores the common obstacles to eating healthy lunches on-the-go and offers practical solutions to overcome them.

1. Time Constraints

Challenge: Limited time to prepare or eat lunch during busy work schedules often leads to opting for fast food or skipping lunch altogether.

Solution:

- **Prep meals in advance**: Use your weekends or evenings to prepare and pack multiple lunches that can be quickly grabbed in the morning.
- **Opt for simple, quick recipes**: Salads, wraps, and bowls can be assembled in minutes and are easy to pack.

2. Limited Options at Work

Challenge: Workplaces often lack healthy food options, or nearby food outlets may offer predominantly high-calorie, processed foods.

Solution:

- **Bring your own lunch**: This is the most reliable method to ensure you have a healthy option.
- **Research local eateries**: Look for cafes or restaurants that offer healthier menus. Many places will list their menus online, allowing you to plan what to order in advance.

3. Social Eating

Challenge: Work lunches and business meetings often occur in restaurants where high-calorie dishes can derail your healthy eating intentions.

Solution:

- **Suggest restaurants with healthy options**: Be proactive in venue selection for business lunches.
- **Choose wisely from the menu**: Opt for dishes with lean proteins and vegetables, and request dressings and sauces on the side.

4. Lack of Proper Storage Facilities

Challenge: Not having access to a refrigerator or microwave at work can limit the types of food you can bring from home.

Solution:

- **Invest in a good, insulated lunch box**: Keep food cold or hot for several hours.
- **Choose non-perishable lunches**: Foods like nuts, whole fruits, and whole-grain crackers are stable at room temperature.

5. Dietary Restrictions

Challenge: Adhering to specific dietary requirements or allergies can complicate finding suitable lunch options while out.

Solution:

- **Label-read and inquire**: Always check labels and ask about ingredients if purchasing prepared food.
- **Prepare allergen-free meals at home**: This ensures that your food meets your dietary needs without the risk of cross-contamination.

Checklist for Eating Healthy Lunches On-the-Go:

- **Meal Prep in Advance**: Spend a part of your weekend preparing lunches for the week.
- **Stock Up on Essentials**: Keep a stash of healthy non-perishable foods in your office, like nuts, seeds, and dried fruits, for emergencies.
- **Hydration**: Always carry a water bottle to avoid sugary drinks.
- **Portable Snacks**: Pack portable, healthy snacks such as carrots with hummus, apples, or yogurt.
- **Mindful Eating**: Take the time to eat away from your desk, focusing on enjoying your meal which can improve digestion and satisfaction.
- **Plan for Outings**: If you know you'll be eating out, plan ahead by looking at the menu online and deciding what healthy options you will choose.

By planning ahead and making conscious choices, you can overcome the common challenges associated with eating a healthy lunch on-the-go or at work. These strategies not only improve your daily nutrition but also enhance your overall health and productivity.

Making healthy swaps at restaurants during the workday

Eating out during the workday is a common scenario for many professionals. While restaurant meals can offer convenience and variety, they often present challenges for those trying to eat healthily.

This chapter outlines effective strategies for making healthier choices when dining out, ensuring you can enjoy a meal that's as good for your body as it is for your taste buds.

1. Salad Dressings and Sauces

Traditional Choice: Creamy dressings and sauces can be high in unhealthy fats and calories. They are often liberally applied to salads, pastas, and entrees, adding significant amounts of hidden calories.

Healthy Swap:

- **Ask for dressings and sauces on the side**: This control allows you to determine the amount you use. Opt for vinaigrette over creamy dressings and request light olive oil and vinegar when available.
- **Choose dishes with clear broths or tomato-based sauces** as opposed to those with cream-based sauces.

2. Entrée Selection

Traditional Choice: Fried foods, dishes prepared with heavy creams, or large cuts of red meat are calorie-dense and can be high in saturated fats.

Healthy Swap:

- **Opt for grilled, steamed, or broiled options**: These cooking methods reduce the amount of fat in the meal and can help maintain the nutritional integrity of the food.
- **Select fish or poultry over red meat**: These are generally lower in saturated fat and calories and can be just as satisfying.

3. Side Dishes

Traditional Choice: Sides like fries, onion rings, or mashed potatoes with gravy are common but add excessive calories and unhealthy fats.

Healthy Swap:

- **Ask for a side salad, steamed vegetables, or a baked potato**: These sides are healthier and can be equally filling. Ensure the vegetables are not cooked with large amounts of butter or oil.

4. Portion Sizes

Traditional Choice: Restaurant portions can be excessively large, encouraging overeating.

Healthy Swap:

- **Share an entrée with a colleague** or ask for a half portion if possible.
- **Consider ordering an appetizer as your main course** or a combination of a salad and an appetizer.

5. Bread Baskets and Starters

Traditional Choice: It's easy to fill up on bread and butter or high-calorie appetizers before the main meal even arrives.

Healthy Swap:

- **Ask the server not to bring the breadbasket to the table**.
- **Choose fresh salads or broth-based soups as a starter**: These are lower in calories and can help you feel full sooner.

Checklist for Healthy Restaurant Swaps During Work Lunches:

- **Preview the Menu Online**: Look at the menu before you go to plan which dishes are healthier options.
- **Watch for Key Words**: Avoid dishes described as "fried," "crispy," or "creamy." Look for "grilled," "baked," "steamed," or "roasted."
- **Special Requests**: Don't be shy about asking for modifications to your meal to make it healthier.
- **Mindful Eating**: Eat slowly and pay attention to your hunger cues, stopping when you're satisfied, not stuffed.
- **Hydrate Smartly**: Stick with water, unsweetened tea, or black coffee instead of sugary beverages or alcoholic drinks during lunch.

By employing these strategies, you can navigate the menu more effectively and make choices that align with your dietary goals. Eating out doesn't have to be a setback in your health journey. With the right approaches, you can enjoy delicious and nutritious meals that fuel your workday without compromising on taste or health.

The top 10 unhealthy lunch foods and their healthy alternatives

Lunchtime can often become a battleground between convenience and nutrition, especially when favorite comfort foods come into play. Here's a guide to the top ten favorite unhealthy lunch foods typically found in the workplace or dining out, along with healthier alternatives to swap in, making your midday meal both satisfying and nutritious.

1. Cheeseburger

Traditional Choice: A cheeseburger can be high in saturated fat, calories, and sodium, especially when topped with bacon or creamy sauces.

Healthy Swap:

- **Opt for a turkey or veggie burger on a whole-grain bun**: Add plenty of veggies like lettuce, tomatoes, and avocado for extra fiber and nutrients without the excess calories.

2. French Fries

Traditional Choice: Deep-fried and salted, French fries are a common side dish that contributes significantly to calorie and fat intake.

Healthy Swap:

- **Choose baked sweet potato fries**: Sweet potatoes are a great source of vitamin A and fiber. Baking reduces fat content significantly.

3. Pizza

Traditional Choice: With its processed meats and high cheese content, traditional pizza is a calorie-dense option with little nutritional benefit.

Healthy Swap:

- **Go for a pizza with a whole-wheat crust, topped with vegetables and a light amount of low-fat cheese**: Consider adding chicken or seafood instead of sausage or pepperoni.

4. Fried Chicken Sandwich

Traditional Choice: Often loaded with mayo and on a white flour bun, fried chicken sandwiches are high in unhealthy fats.

Healthy Swap:

- **Choose a grilled chicken sandwich**: Opt for mustard or a yogurt-based sauce instead of mayo, and pick a whole-grain bun.

5. Nachos

Traditional Choice: Laden with cheese and often sour cream, nachos are high in fat and calories.

Healthy Swap:

- **Create a nacho bowl with baked tortilla chips, black beans, salsa, avocado, and a sprinkle of cheese**: This version offers more fiber and healthy fats.

6. Cream-based Soups

Traditional Choice: Soups like clam chowder or broccoli cheese soup are often high in saturated fat and calories.

Healthy Swap:

- **Select broth-based soups**: Options like vegetable or chicken noodle are satisfying but lower in calories and fat.

7. Deli Meat Sandwich

Traditional Choice: Processed deli meats can be high in sodium and preservatives.

Healthy Swap:

- **Use roasted turkey or chicken breast**: Pile on the veggies and swap out mayo for hummus or avocado for a healthier spread.

8. Burritos

Traditional Choice: Large flour tortillas and fillings like refried beans and rice can make burritos calorie-dense and high in carbs.

Healthy Swap:

- **Opt for a burrito bowl with brown rice, beans, fresh salsa, and vegetables**: Skip the cheese and sour cream and add extra lettuce and tomatoes.

9. Potato Chips

Traditional Choice: A common side item, potato chips are high in sodium and trans fats.

Healthy Swap:

- **Choose baked chips or veggie chips**: Alternatively, bring a side of raw veggies like carrot sticks or cucumber with hummus for crunch.

10. Carbonated Soft Drinks

Traditional Choice: Sugary sodas are high in calories and contribute to tooth decay and poor health.

Healthy Swap:

- **Drink sparkling water with a splash of fruit juice**: This provides the fizzy satisfaction with fewer calories and no added sugars.

Checklist for Healthy Lunch Swaps:

- Choose lean proteins over fatty or fried options.
- Opt for whole grains instead of refined grains.
- Increase vegetable intake to boost fiber and reduce calorie density.
- Select healthy fats like avocado and nuts over saturated fats.
- Stay hydrated with water or unsweetened beverages.

By substituting these healthier alternatives, you not only reduce your caloric and fat intake but also enhance your lunch with nutrients that promote long-term health and energy levels throughout the workday.

Preparing and packing powerful, portable lunches

Whether you're rushing between meetings or need a quick meal before a workout, having a portable lunch that's both nutritious and convenient can make a significant difference in maintaining your health and energy levels.

This chapter offers strategies for preparing and packing lunches that are tasty, nutritious, and easy to carry, ensuring you never have to rely on less healthy options.

1. Choose the Right Containers

Principle: Proper storage is key to keeping your meals fresh and appetizing. Invest in high-quality, durable, and leak-proof containers. Bento boxes and insulated lunch bags can help maintain food temperature and quality.

Checklist:

- Use airtight containers to keep food fresh.
- Choose containers that are microwave safe if you need to reheat the meal.
- Have a variety of sizes for different components of your lunch.

2. Focus on Macro and Micronutrient Balance

Principle: A balanced lunch that includes a good mix of protein, carbohydrates, and fats will keep you full and energized. Don't forget to include a variety of fruits and vegetables to get a range of vitamins and minerals.

Checklist:

- Include a protein source such as chicken, fish, beans, or tofu.
- Add complex carbohydrates like quinoa, whole-grain bread, or sweet potatoes.
- Incorporate healthy fats from sources like avocados, nuts, or seeds.
- Pack colorful vegetables and fruits to maximize nutrient intake.

3. Plan Ahead

Principle: Advance planning is the secret to stress-free and healthy lunch packing. Prepare meals that can be made in bulk and used throughout the week, or use leftovers creatively.

Checklist:

- Dedicate time for meal planning and grocery shopping each week.
- Prepare and cook in bulk where possible.
- Portion out meals right after cooking to save time in the mornings.

4. Keep it Simple and Varied

Principle: Simple meals are easier to prepare and pack. However, variety is essential to avoid boredom and ensure a range of nutrients.

Checklist:

- Rotate the types of proteins, veggies, and carbs weekly.
- Use different herbs and spices to change the flavor profiles without adding calories.
- Experiment with various types of cuisine for diversity, like Mediterranean one week and Mexican the next.

5. Quick Assembly Options

Principle: Some days are busier than others. Having components on hand that can be quickly assembled into a meal can save the day.

Checklist:

- Keep washed and chopped veggies in the fridge for quick grabs.
- Have portions of cooked grains like rice or pasta ready to use.
- Stock a variety of canned or pre-cooked proteins like beans, lentils, or tuna for convenience.

6. Snacks and Hydration

Principle: Healthy snacks and proper hydration are crucial to keep you alert and prevent overeating later in the day.

Checklist:

- Pack fresh or dried fruit, nuts, yogurt, or whole-grain crackers for snacks.
- Include a reusable water bottle to ensure you stay hydrated throughout the day.
- Consider unsweetened tea or coffee if you need a caffeine boost.

Conclusion

Preparing and packing your lunches not only saves money but also ensures you're fueled by nutrient-rich foods that support your health goals. By incorporating these strategies and making lunch preparation an integral part of your routine, you can enjoy delicious, homemade meals that are perfectly tailored to your dietary needs, even on your busiest days.

Chapter 5: Snacks - Smart Munching

Identifying unhealthy snack habits

Snacking can either be a pitfall in one's diet or a bridge between meals that supports energy levels and nutritional intake. Unfortunately, unhealthy snacking habits are easy to develop and can sabotage weight management and health goals.

This chapter focuses on identifying common unhealthy snacking habits and offers strategies to correct them.

1. Snacking Out of Boredom or Stress

Problem: Many people turn to snacks not because of hunger but due to emotional triggers like boredom, stress, or fatigue. This can lead to overeating and the consumption of high-calorie, nutrient-poor snacks.

Checklist:

- Recognize emotional eating triggers.
- Develop non-eating methods to address these emotions, such as taking a walk, doing a quick workout, or engaging in a hobby.
- Keep unhealthy snacks out of reach, and don't buy them during your regular shopping.

2. Choosing High-Sugar, High-Fat Snacks

Problem: Snacks such as chips, cookies, and candy are high in sugars and unhealthy fats but low in essential nutrients. Regular consumption can lead to health issues such as obesity, diabetes, and heart disease.

Checklist:

- Read labels to avoid snacks with high amounts of added sugars and saturated fats.
- Replace sugary snacks with fruits or yogurt topped with nuts for added sweetness plus fiber and protein.
- Opt for air-popped popcorn or homemade trail mix instead of chips and other fried items.

3. Mindless Eating

Problem: Eating while distracted (e.g., eating while working or watching TV) can lead to consuming more calories than needed as it's easy to lose track of how much has been eaten.

Checklist:

- Always portion out snacks instead of eating directly from the package.
- Avoid snacking while distracted by screens or work; instead, take deliberate breaks to enjoy your snack.
- Use smaller plates or bowls to control portion sizes.

4. Not Incorporating Variety

Problem: Repeating the same snacks can lead to nutritional gaps. Variety in snacks can provide a wider range of nutrients and prevent boredom, which might lead to seeking out less healthy options.

Checklist:

- Rotate your snacks weekly to include a variety of food groups.
- Incorporate different types of fruits, vegetables, nuts, seeds, whole grains, and lean proteins.
- Try new recipes for homemade snacks that include multiple nutrient-dense ingredients.

5. Late-Night Snacking

Problem: Eating late at night, especially right before bed, can disrupt sleep and lead to weight gain. These snacks tend to be high in calories and low in nutritional value.

Checklist:

- Set a cutoff time for eating, ideally two to three hours before bed.
- Choose light snacks if needed, such as a small serving of almonds or a piece of fruit.
- Evaluate if your dinner is filling and nutritious enough to prevent late-night hunger.

6. Relying on Convenience Store or Vending Machine Snacks

Problem: Snacks from convenience stores or vending machines typically lack nutritional value and are high in sugar, salt, and fats.

Checklist:

- Prepare snacks in advance to take with you, such as cut veggies, fruits, or whole-grain crackers.
- Keep a stash of healthy snacks at your workplace, such as in a desk drawer or fridge.
- When you must buy from a vending machine, opt for the healthiest option available, such as nuts or a granola bar.

Conclusion

By recognizing and modifying these unhealthy snacking habits, you can significantly improve your diet quality.

Healthier snacking is about preparation, variety, and mindfulness, which can lead to better overall health and more effective weight management. Taking the time to assess and adjust your snacking habits can lead to lasting positive changes in your eating patterns.

Healthier alternatives to chips, cookies, and other common snacks

Snacking is an integral part of daily eating habits for many people, but commonly chosen snacks like chips and cookies are often loaded with unhealthy fats, sugars, and excessive calories. Opting for healthier alternatives can contribute significantly to improved nutrition and overall health. This chapter provides practical, healthier snack options that satisfy cravings without compromising nutritional goals.

1. Instead of Potato Chips

Traditional Choice: Potato chips are high in saturated fats and sodium, and they offer little nutritional value.

Healthier Swap:

- **Kale or seaweed chips**: These are low in calories and provide vitamins and minerals.
- **Air-popped popcorn**: This whole grain is high in fiber and can be seasoned with a minimal amount of salt or other spices for flavor without the fat.
- **Vegetable chips made from carrots, sweet potatoes, or zucchini**: When baked, these chips offer a satisfying crunch with the added benefits of fiber and nutrients.

2. Instead of Cookies

Traditional Choice: Cookies are typically high in sugar, refined flours, and unhealthy fats.

Healthier Swap:

- **Oatmeal cookies made with whole grains, nuts, and natural sweeteners**: These provide fiber, protein, and are lower in sugar.
- **Fruit slices with nut butter**: This snack offers a sweet taste with the added benefits of protein and healthy fats from the nut butter.
- **Homemade energy bars**: Combine oats, dried fruit, honey, and nuts for a sweet treat that's nutritious and energy-boosting.

3. Instead of Candy

Traditional Choice: Candy is almost purely sugar with little to no nutritional value, contributing to tooth decay and potential weight gain.

Healthier Swap:

- **Dried fruit with no added sugar**: Offers natural sweetness along with fiber and nutrients.
- **Dark chocolate with a high percentage of cocoa**: Contains antioxidants and can satisfy chocolate cravings with a smaller portion.
- **Frozen grapes or berries**: These provide a candy-like texture and natural sweetness, with the added benefit of vitamins and antioxidants.

4. Instead of Creamy Dips

Traditional Choice: Dips like ranch or onion dip are often calorie-dense and high in unhealthy fats.

Healthier Swap:

- **Hummus or guacamole**: Both are rich in nutrients and healthy fats. They pair well with raw vegetables for a filling snack.
- **Greek yogurt dip**: Mix Greek yogurt with herbs and spices for a protein-rich alternative to sour cream dips.

5. Instead of Sugary Beverages

Traditional Choice: Sodas and fruit juices are high in sugars and often contain little to no actual fruit juice, offering empty calories without satisfying hunger.

Healthier Swap:

- **Infused water**: Add slices of fruits or cucumbers to water for a refreshing and hydrating drink.
- **Herbal tea, hot or iced**: Provides hydration without added sugar. If sweetness is desired, a small amount of honey can be added.
- **Sparkling water with a splash of juice**: Offers the fizzy texture of soda but with significantly fewer calories and sugars.

Checklist for Choosing Healthier Snacks:

- Always check labels for hidden sugars, unhealthy fats, and sodium, even in products marketed as healthy.
- Prepare snacks at home to control ingredients and portions.
- Include a variety of textures and flavors to keep snacking interesting and satisfying.
- Keep portion sizes in check to manage calorie intake, even when snacking on healthier options.
- Store healthy snacks at eye level in your pantry or fridge to make them the easy choice.

By replacing common unhealthy snacks with these healthier alternatives, you can enjoy the benefits of snacking without the guilt. These swaps help maintain energy levels, manage hunger, and contribute to a balanced diet.

Ideas for satisfying and energizing snacks

Snacks play a crucial role in maintaining energy throughout the day, preventing overeating at mealtimes, and supplying the body with essential nutrients. However, choosing the right snacks can be challenging. This chapter provides ideas for snacks that are both satisfying and energizing, along with practical tips to incorporate them into your daily routine.

1. High-Protein Snacks

Benefit: Protein is essential for building and repairing tissues and maintaining muscle mass. It also helps you feel full longer, which can prevent overeating.

Snack Ideas:

- **Greek yogurt with a handful of nuts or seeds**: This combination provides protein, healthy fats, and a bit of crunch.
- **Cottage cheese with pineapple or berries**: Cottage cheese is high in protein, and fruits add a natural sweetness and fiber.
- **Hard-boiled eggs**: They are portable, packed with protein, and can be seasoned with a pinch of salt and pepper or paprika for extra flavor.

2. Whole Grains

Benefit: Whole grains provide sustained energy due to their high fiber content, which helps regulate blood sugar levels.

Snack Ideas:

- **Air-popped popcorn**: Toss it with a little olive oil and a sprinkle of nutritional yeast or sea salt for flavor.
- **Whole-grain crackers with avocado mash**: Avocado provides heart-healthy fats, while whole-grain crackers are a good source of fiber.
- **Homemade granola bars**: Combine oats, honey, nuts, and dried fruits for a sweet and filling snack.

3. Fresh Fruits and Vegetables

Benefit: Fruits and vegetables are rich in vitamins, minerals, and antioxidants that contribute to overall health and help fight fatigue.

Snack Ideas:

- **Carrot and celery sticks with hummus**: This snack packs fiber and protein, keeping you full and energized.
- **An apple or banana with almond butter**: The fruit provides natural sugars and fiber for energy, while almond butter adds protein and healthy fats.
- **Seasonal berries or grapes**: Easy to eat on the go, berries and grapes provide hydration and a quick energy boost.

4. Nuts and Seeds

Benefit: Nuts and seeds are excellent sources of healthy fats, proteins, and fiber. They also contain vitamins and minerals like vitamin E, magnesium, and zinc.

Snack Ideas:

- **A handful of mixed nuts or trail mix**: Choose raw or dry-roasted varieties without added salts or sugars.
- **Pumpkin or sunflower seeds**: These are high in protein and fiber, which help sustain energy levels.
- **Chia pudding**: Made with chia seeds and almond milk, this snack can be flavored with vanilla or cocoa for a dessert-like treat.

5. Energy Balls

Benefit: Energy balls are a dense source of nutrients, providing a balanced mix of protein, healthy fats, and carbohydrates.

Snack Ideas:

- **Date and nut energy balls**: Blend dates with nuts like almonds or walnuts and roll in coconut flakes for a sweet, energizing snack.
- **Oat and peanut butter balls**: Mix rolled oats, peanut butter, honey, and mini dark chocolate chips for a satisfying bite.

Checklist for Preparing Snacks:

- Keep your pantry and refrigerator stocked with healthy snacking ingredients.
- Prepare snacks in advance to grab and go on busy days.
- Portion out snacks to avoid overeating.
- Keep a variety at hand to suit different moods and hunger levels.
- Include a good balance of macronutrients (protein, fats, carbohydrates) to maximize satiety and energy.

By choosing the right snacks and preparing them ahead of time, you can ensure that you have quick access to energy-boosting and nutritious options throughout your day. This approach not only helps maintain steady energy levels but also contributes to a more balanced diet, enhancing overall health and well-being.

Chapter 6: Dinner - ending the day on a high note

Common unhealthy dinner components and their healthy substitutes

Dinner is a critical meal that can either support your day's nutrition or undermine it significantly. Many traditional dinner components, though popular, are not always the healthiest options. This chapter explores common unhealthy dinner components often found in typical meals and provides practical, healthier alternatives to incorporate into your evening routine.

1. Refined Carbohydrates

Traditional Choice: White rice, white pasta, and white bread are common dinner staples that offer limited nutritional value because they lack fiber and cause rapid spikes in blood sugar levels.

Healthy Substitute:

- **Whole grains such as brown rice, quinoa, or whole-wheat pasta**: These alternatives provide more fiber, which helps in digestion and sustained energy release.
- **Cauliflower rice or spiralized vegetables**: For a lower-carbohydrate option, these provide additional nutrients and fewer calories than their refined counterparts.

2. Creamy Sauces

Traditional Choice: Sauces like Alfredo or heavy cream-based gravies are high in saturated fats and calories.

Healthy Substitute:

- **Tomato-based sauces or pesto**: These alternatives offer flavor with fewer calories and beneficial nutrients like lycopene in tomatoes.
- **Greek yogurt or pureed avocado**: These can be used to create creamy textures without unhealthy fats.

3. Fatty Cuts of Meat

Traditional Choice: Items like ribeye steaks or pork chops are often rich in saturated fat.

Healthy Substitute:

- **Lean proteins like chicken breast, turkey, or fish**: These meats are lower in fat but high in protein.
- **Plant-based proteins such as lentils, chickpeas, or tofu**: These provide fiber and protein without the saturated fat.

4. Deep-Fried Foods

Traditional Choice: Fried foods are a popular dinner choice but are high in unhealthy fats and calories.

Healthy Substitute:

- **Baked or air-fried options**: Achieve a similar texture and taste without the health drawbacks of deep frying.
- **Grilling or broiling**: These cooking methods reduce fat content while adding flavor.

5. High-Sodium Side Dishes

Traditional Choice: Sides like canned beans or instant mashed potatoes often contain high levels of sodium.

Healthy Substitute:

- **Home-prepared sides with fresh ingredients**: Control the amount of salt added.
- **Use herbs and spices instead of salt**: Enhance flavor naturally without increasing sodium intake.

6. Sugary Desserts

Traditional Choice: Desserts are typically loaded with sugars and fats, contributing to excessive calorie intake.

Healthy Substitute:

- **Fresh fruit or fruit-based desserts**: Offer natural sweetness along with fiber and vitamins.
- **Dark chocolate**: Provides antioxidants with less sugar than milk chocolate.

Checklist for Healthier Dinner Choices:

- Plan your meals to include a balance of protein, carbohydrates, and healthy fats.
- Choose whole grain or vegetable-based alternatives to refined carbohydrates.
- Opt for cooking methods like baking, grilling, or steaming instead of frying.
- Prepare sauces and sides at home to control ingredients and avoid unnecessary fats and salts.
- Incorporate a variety of vegetables to increase fiber and nutrient intake.
- Select desserts that provide nutritional benefits, like those based on fruits or containing minimal added sugars.

By replacing unhealthy dinner components with these healthier alternatives, you can enjoy a nutritious meal that supports your well-being without sacrificing flavor. Making these swaps helps maintain a balanced diet and can lead to better health outcomes.

Swaps for popular dishes from various cuisines

Exploring different cuisines is a delightful way to enjoy meals, but many popular dishes in international cuisine can be high in calories, fats, and sodium. This chapter offers healthier alternatives and swaps for popular dishes from Italian, Mexican, and Asian cuisines, ensuring you can savor global flavors without compromising your health goals.

1. Italian Cuisine

Traditional Choice: Dishes like lasagna, fettuccine Alfredo, and pizza are staples of Italian cuisine but often come loaded with cheese, creamy sauces, and refined carbs.

Healthy Substitute:

- **Whole grain or legume-based pasta**: Swap traditional pasta for whole grain, lentil, or chickpea pasta to increase fiber and protein content.
- **Light homemade sauces**: Use tomato-based sauces and add vegetables like spinach or mushrooms for a nutritional boost. For a creamy texture, blend cottage cheese or use Greek yogurt.
- **Grilled vegetable pizza on a cauliflower crust**: Top with a small amount of low-fat cheese and plenty of vegetables for a satisfying but lighter pizza.

2. Mexican Cuisine

Traditional Choice: While flavorful, many Mexican dishes such as burritos and nachos are often prepared with excessive cheese, sour cream, and fried tortillas.

Healthy Substitute:

- **Use whole wheat or corn tortillas**: These are healthier than flour tortillas and provide more fiber.
- **Lean proteins and beans**: Choose grilled chicken, fish, or black beans as main protein sources for tacos and burritos instead of fried meats or refried beans.
- **Salsa and avocado**: Opt for salsa and avocado instead of cheese and sour cream to add flavor and healthy fats.

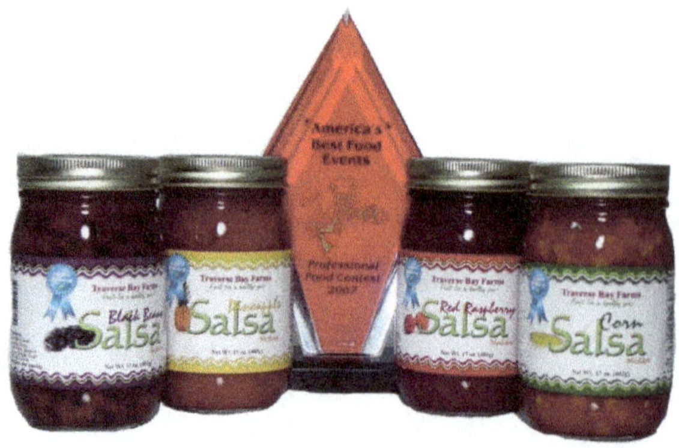

  Check out Traverse Bay Farms all-natural, nationally award-winning salsa with ZERO fat. They have cherry, black bean, corn, peach pineapple, red raspberry and more.

3. Asian Cuisine

Traditional Choice: Asian dishes can sometimes be high in sodium and sugar, particularly in sauces used in Chinese takeout or fried Japanese tempura.

Healthy Substitute:

- **Sushi with brown rice or no rice**: Opt for sashimi, naruto rolls (wrapped in cucumber), or sushi made with brown rice to lower the glycemic index.
- **Stir-fried or steamed dishes**: Choose stir-fries or steamed dishes with lots of vegetables and lean proteins like tofu, chicken, or shrimp. Ask for sauce on the side to control the amount used.
- **Low-sodium soy sauce**: Use low-sodium soy sauce in moderation to reduce salt intake.

Checklist for Making Healthier Choices in International Cuisines:

- Choose dishes that feature a variety of vegetables to increase your nutrient intake.
- Opt for whole grains over refined grains where possible (brown rice, whole wheat pasta).
- Select lean protein options to reduce intake of saturated fat.
- Request sauces and dressings on the side to control how much you consume.
- Watch portion sizes, especially when dining out, as restaurant portions can be quite large.
- Avoid dishes that are described as "fried," "breaded," or "creamy," as these are usually higher in unhealthy fats and calories.
- Experiment with making your favorite international dishes at home where you can control the ingredients and cooking methods.

By integrating these swaps and suggestions into your meals, you can enjoy a diverse range of international flavors while maintaining a balanced and health-conscious diet. These healthier versions not only cater to your taste buds but also contribute positively to your overall health by reducing unnecessary fats, sugars, and sodium.

Cooking methods that preserve and enhance nutritional value

The way we cook our food can significantly impact its nutritional content. Some cooking methods can degrade vitamins and minerals, while others enhance the availability of these nutrients and the overall health benefits of the meals we eat. This chapter discusses various cooking techniques that not only preserve but can also boost the nutritional value of food, ensuring that every meal is as healthful as possible.

1. Steaming

Benefit: Steaming is one of the best methods for preserving the integrity of vitamins and minerals, particularly water-soluble vitamins like vitamin C and B vitamins, which are prone to degradation when exposed to heat. Steaming minimizes contact with cooking water, preventing these nutrients from being leached out.

Healthy Applications:

- **Vegetables**: Steaming vegetables like broccoli, spinach, and carrots enhances their natural flavors without the need for excess oil or salt.
- **Fish**: Steaming fish preserves its delicate texture and nutrients like omega-3 fatty acids.

2. Poaching

Benefit: Poaching involves cooking food at a lower temperature than boiling, using gentle heat. This method is excellent for preserving the tenderness of food and preventing the loss of some nutrients that can occur at higher temperatures.

Healthy Applications:

- **Eggs**: Poached eggs retain all their protein without needing added fats for cooking.
- **Poultry and fish**: Poaching can be used to cook these proteins thoroughly while keeping them moist and flavorful.

3. Grilling

Benefit: Grilling foods enhances flavor through caramelization and can be a low-fat cooking method if excess marinades and fatty meats are avoided. It also helps vegetables and meats retain antioxidants and vitamins that might be lost during other cooking methods.

Healthy Applications:

- **Vegetables**: Grill a variety of vegetables with a minimal brush of olive oil for a flavorful, nutrient-rich side dish.
- **Lean meats**: Grill chicken, fish, or lean cuts of beef to reduce fat content while adding robust flavor.

4. Baking or Roasting

Benefit: Baking or roasting in an oven can concentrate flavors and naturally caramelize food's exterior, adding to its palatability without additional fats. This method also preserves nutrients by using dry heat, which is less likely to cause nutrient loss than boiling or frying.

Healthy Applications:

- **Root vegetables**: Baking or roasting carrots, sweet potatoes, and beets can enhance their natural sweetness.
- **Whole grains and legumes**: Prepare dishes like baked falafel or roasted chickpeas for a crunchy, nutritious snack.

5. Sautéing

Benefit: Sautéing quickly cooks foods at a relatively high heat with a small amount of oil or water, preserving texture, flavor, and nutrients, especially when compared to deep frying.

Healthy Applications:

- **Leafy greens**: Quickly sauté spinach or kale with garlic in olive oil for a fast and healthy side.
- **Mushrooms and onions**: Sautéing these can bring out rich flavors suitable for enhancing main dishes.

Checklist for Nutrient-Preserving Cooking:

- Use as little water as possible when cooking vegetables to prevent nutrient loss.
- Cook foods for the shortest time necessary to maintain nutrients.
- Use healthy fats like olive oil sparingly to enhance flavor without adding excessive calories.
- Incorporate a variety of spices and herbs to boost flavor and nutritional value without adding salt.
- Choose fresh, local ingredients to maximize flavor and nutritional content.
- Practice proper food handling and storage to preserve freshness and nutrient quality before cooking.

By choosing cooking methods that enhance and preserve nutritional value, you can ensure that your meals are not only delicious but also contribute positively to your health. These techniques allow you to enjoy the natural tastes and benefits of your food, making every meal a nourishing experience.

Chapter 7: Desserts - sweet solutions

The impact of sugar and unhealthy fats in traditional desserts

Desserts are a beloved part of many cultures' dining experiences, offering a sweet end to meals. However, traditional desserts often contain high amounts of sugars and unhealthy fats, which can have significant negative impacts on health when consumed frequently. This chapter explores the health consequences of these ingredients and offers guidance on how to enjoy desserts in a healthier way.

1. The Impact of High Sugar Intake

Health Effects:

- **Increased Risk of Obesity**: Sugars, especially added sugars found in desserts, contribute to excessive calorie intake, a leading factor in obesity (Malik et al., 2010).
- **Dental Problems**: Frequent consumption of sugary desserts can lead to dental caries and tooth decay.
- **Higher Risk of Type 2 Diabetes**: Regular consumption of high-sugar foods can lead to insulin resistance, eventually increasing the risk of developing type 2 diabetes (Hu & Malik, 2010).
- **Cardiovascular Disease**: Studies have linked high sugar intake to increased risks of high blood pressure, inflammation, and higher levels of harmful cholesterol (Stanhope, 2016).

2. The Impact of Unhealthy Fats

Health Effects:

- **Increased LDL Cholesterol**: Trans fats and saturated fats found in many desserts can raise LDL (bad) cholesterol levels, contributing to the buildup of plaques in arteries and increasing heart disease risk.
- **Weight Gain**: High-fat foods are calorically dense and can contribute to unwanted weight gain if not balanced with overall calorie intake.
- **Increased Risk of Heart Disease**: Consuming high levels of unhealthy fats is linked to cardiovascular disease due to their effects on heart function and blood lipids.

Strategies for Healthier Dessert Choices

Checklist:

- **Reduce Portion Sizes**: Opt for smaller portions to enjoy desserts without consuming excessive amounts of sugar and fat.
- **Choose Natural Sweeteners**: Use fruits, honey, or maple syrup instead of refined sugar to sweeten desserts, which can offer additional nutrients and less impact on blood glucose levels.
- **Opt for Healthier Fats**: Use unsaturated fats like olive oil or avocado oil in place of butter or shortening when possible.
- **Incorporate Whole Grains**: Replace refined flour with whole grains like oat flour or whole wheat flour to add fiber and nutrients.
- **Add Fruits and Nuts**: Include fresh or dried fruits and nuts to provide fiber, vitamins, and healthy fats, enhancing the nutritional profile of desserts.
- **Moderation is Key**: Enjoy desserts as an occasional treat rather than a daily indulgence to keep sugar and fat intake in check.

Educational Tips:

- **Read Labels Carefully**: When purchasing store-bought desserts, read the nutritional information to avoid high-sugar and high-fat products.
- **Be Aware of Liquid Calories**: Remember that sugary drinks can be just as detrimental as solid desserts. Opt for water, unsweetened tea, or coffee to accompany your dessert.
- **Practice Mindful Eating**: Savor your dessert slowly to increase satisfaction and reduce the likelihood of overeating.

By understanding the impacts of sugar and unhealthy fats found in traditional desserts and making informed choices, it is possible to enjoy these treats in a way that is mindful of health and well-being. Implementing these strategies can allow you to appreciate desserts without compromising your health objectives, blending indulgence with a balanced approach to eating.

Healthier alternatives to ice cream, cakes, and pies

Desserts like ice cream, cakes, and pies are staples in many diets, but they often come loaded with sugars and fats that can detract from health goals. This chapter offers creative, healthier alternatives to these traditional desserts, allowing you to indulge your sweet tooth without the guilt.

1. Healthier Ice Cream Alternatives

Traditional ice cream is high in sugar and fat, which can contribute to weight gain and associated health issues.

Healthier Swaps:

- **Frozen yogurt**: Opt for frozen yogurt as a lower-fat alternative to traditional ice cream. Look for versions without added sugars.
- **Banana ice cream**: Blend frozen bananas until smooth to create a creamy, naturally sweet ice cream alternative. Add flavors like vanilla or cocoa powder for variety.
- **Sorbet**: Made from churned fruit and water, sorbet is a light, refreshing dessert that skips the dairy and reduces fat content.

2. Healthier Cake Alternatives

Traditional cakes are often made with refined sugars and flours, contributing to rapid spikes in blood sugar.

Healthier Swaps:

- **Flourless cakes**: Use almond or coconut flour instead of white flour for a gluten-free, lower-glycemic alternative.
- **Add fruits and vegetables**: Incorporate mashed bananas, applesauce, or grated vegetables like carrots and zucchini to add natural sweetness and moisture without extra fat.
- **Reduce sugar**: Cut the amount of sugar in recipes and enhance sweetness with natural options like pureed dates or applesauce.

3. Healthier Pie Alternatives

Pies, while delicious, are typically made with sugar-heavy fillings and buttery crusts.

Healthier Swaps:

- **Whole grain or nut-based crusts**: Replace traditional pie crusts with ones made from whole grains, oats, or ground nuts for added fiber and nutrients.
- **Lighter fillings**: Use fresh fruit for fillings, lightly sweetened with honey or maple syrup instead of sugar. Consider using Greek yogurt for creamy pies.
- **Mini pies**: Bake smaller portions to help control serving sizes and reduce overall calorie intake.

Checklist for Creating Healthier Desserts:

- **Choose natural sweeteners**: Opt for honey, maple syrup, or ripe fruits to sweeten desserts naturally.
- **Use healthy fats**: Incorporate avocados, nut butters, or olive oil instead of butter.
- **Incorporate whole grains and nuts**: Use oats, almond meal, or whole wheat flour to add fiber and nutrients.
- **Experiment with dairy-free alternatives**: Try coconut milk, almond milk, or cashew cream for creamy textures without the dairy.
- **Control portion sizes**: Prepare desserts in individual cups or mini pans to keep portions in check.
- **Focus on fruits**: Make fruits the star in desserts, whether in raw, baked, or pureed form, to capitalize on their natural sweetness and health benefits.
- **Be mindful of toppings**: Choose toppings like dark chocolate, toasted nuts, or a sprinkle of cinnamon instead of sugary glazes or whipped cream.

By implementing these alternatives and tips, you can enjoy delicious desserts that satisfy your cravings while also fitting into a healthy eating plan. These swaps not only reduce the intake of unhealthy ingredients but also enhance your diet with more nutritious elements, making each dessert not just a treat but a beneficial part of your meals.

Recipes for delicious, guilt-free treats

Indulging in a sweet treat doesn't have to mean derailing your healthy eating habits. With a few smart swaps and creative recipes, you can enjoy desserts that are both delicious and nutritious. This chapter provides recipes for guilt-free treats that use healthy ingredients and preparation methods to keep them lower in sugar and fat but high in flavor.

1. Avocado Chocolate Mousse

Ingredients:

- 2 ripe avocados, peeled and pitted
- 1/4 cup cocoa powder
- 1/4 cup pure maple syrup or honey
- 1/2 teaspoon vanilla extract
- A pinch of salt
- 1/4 cup unsweetened almond milk

Instructions:

1. Combine all ingredients in a blender or food processor.
2. Blend until smooth, scraping down the sides as necessary.
3. Adjust sweetness with more maple syrup or honey if desired.
4. Chill in the refrigerator for at least an hour before serving.
5. Serve with a sprinkle of sea salt or fresh raspberries for an extra touch.

This mousse is rich in healthy fats from the avocado and antioxidants from the cocoa, making it a satisfying dessert that's good for your heart and skin.

2. Oatmeal Banana Cookies

Ingredients:

- 2 ripe bananas, mashed
- 1 cup rolled oats
- 1/4 cup chopped nuts (walnuts or almonds)
- 1/4 cup dried cranberries or raisins
- 1/2 teaspoon cinnamon
- A pinch of salt

Instructions:

1. Preheat the oven to 350°F (175°C).
2. In a large bowl, mix all the ingredients together until well combined.
3. Drop spoonfuls of the mixture onto a baking sheet lined with parchment paper.
4. Flatten each mound slightly with the back of a spoon.
5. Bake for 12-15 minutes or until the edges are golden.
6. Let cool on the baking sheet before transferring to a wire rack to cool completely.

These cookies are naturally sweetened by bananas and offer a great source of fiber from oats and a protein boost from nuts.

3. Coconut Yogurt Parfait

Ingredients:

- 1 cup unsweetened coconut yogurt
- 1/2 cup mixed berries (such as blueberries, strawberries, and raspberries)
- 1/4 cup granola
- 1 tablespoon chia seeds
- Honey or maple syrup (optional)

Instructions:

1. In a glass or jar, layer half of the coconut yogurt at the bottom.
2. Add a layer of mixed berries followed by a sprinkle of granola and chia seeds.
3. Repeat the layers until all ingredients are used up.
4. Drizzle with a little honey or maple syrup if a sweeter taste is desired.
5. Serve immediately or chill in the refrigerator until ready to eat.

This parfait is an excellent source of probiotics, antioxidants, and fiber, making it a perfect start to your day or a refreshing snack.

Checklist for Preparing Guilt-Free Treats:

- Use natural sweeteners like fruits, honey, or maple syrup instead of refined sugar.
- Choose whole grains and nuts to add texture and nutrients.
- Incorporate healthy fats such as avocados or nut butters to enrich flavor and consistency.
- Opt for dairy alternatives like coconut or almond milk to reduce calories and add variety.
- Remember portion control, even with healthier options.
- Be creative with spices like cinnamon, nutmeg, or vanilla to enhance flavor without added sugar.

These recipes prove that with the right ingredients and techniques, you can create treats that satisfy your sweet tooth without compromising your health. Enjoy these guilt-free desserts that will delight your palate and support your wellness journey.

Chapter 8: Beverages - drink to your health

Common unhealthy beverages and their effects on health

Beverages can either be a refreshing nourishment for the body or a hidden source of excessive sugars and unwanted chemicals. Many popular drinks, such as sodas, energy drinks, and some types of coffee beverages, contribute to various health issues when consumed regularly. This chapter delves into the most common unhealthy beverages, their potential health impacts, and provides a checklist for making healthier choices.

1. Sugary Soft Drinks

Health Effects:

- **Obesity**: Soft drinks are high in calories and sugars and offer no nutritional value, contributing significantly to weight gain when consumed frequently (Malik et al., 2010).
- **Type 2 Diabetes**: Regular consumption of sugary beverages is linked to a higher risk of developing type 2 diabetes due to constant spikes in blood sugar levels (Hu & Malik, 2010).
- **Tooth Decay**: The high sugar content and acids in soft drinks promote tooth enamel erosion and cavities.

2. Energy Drinks

Health Effects:

- **Cardiovascular Problems**: Energy drinks contain high levels of caffeine and other stimulants that can increase heart rate and blood pressure, potentially leading to heart rhythm disturbances or other serious heart issues (Fletcher et al., 2017).
- **Sleep Disturbances**: The excessive caffeine in these drinks can disrupt sleep patterns, leading to sleep deprivation and related problems like difficulty concentrating and mood swings.
- **Addiction and Dependence**: Regular consumption can lead to caffeine addiction, characterized by a dependence on these drinks to function normally.

3. Pre-Made Alcoholic Cocktails

Health Effects:

- **Liver Damage**: Excessive alcohol consumption can lead to a range of liver problems, including fatty liver, hepatitis, and cirrhosis.
- **Weight Gain**: Alcoholic beverages are calorie-dense, and pre-made cocktails often include additional sugars, contributing to increased caloric intake.
- **Increased Risk of Chronic Diseases**: Long-term consumption increases the risk of developing heart disease, stroke, and certain types of cancer.

4. Creamy Coffee Drinks

Health Effects:

- **High Caloric Content**: Many popular coffee drinks include high amounts of syrups, sugars, and cream, leading to high calorie counts that can contribute to weight gain.
- **Sugar Spikes**: The high sugar content can cause quick spikes and crashes in blood sugar levels, leading to energy slumps and potential insulin sensitivity issues over time.
- **Poor Nutrient Density**: These beverages often displace more nutritious options, contributing to nutrient deficiencies.

Checklist for Choosing Healthier Beverages:

- **Read Labels**: Always check the nutritional content of beverages, focusing on sugar and calorie content.
- **Choose Water First**: Prioritize water intake throughout the day to ensure proper hydration.
- **Opt for Unsweetened Options**: Choose tea or coffee without added sugars or flavored syrups.
- **Limit Alcohol Intake**: Consume alcohol in moderation and opt for simpler mixed drinks like a gin and tonic instead of sugary cocktails.
- **Avoid Drinking Calories**: Stay aware of the caloric content of beverages and avoid using drinks as a substitute for nourishing meals.
- **DIY Drinks**: Prepare homemade versions of your favorite beverages so you can control the ingredients and reduce unwanted sugars and additives.

By understanding the impacts of common unhealthy beverages and implementing the suggestions from the checklist, you can make informed choices that minimize risks to your health while still enjoying a variety of satisfying drinks. Making simple swaps and choosing water or other healthy alternatives can significantly benefit your overall wellness.

Smart Swaps for soda, alcohol, and high-calorie coffee drinks

Many popular beverages such as soda, alcoholic drinks, and specialty coffee beverages contribute significantly to daily calorie intake, often without providing any nutritional benefits. This chapter explores healthier alternatives to these drinks, helping you to reduce sugar and calorie consumption while still enjoying satisfying beverages.

1. Swaps for Soda

Traditional Choice: Regular sodas are high in added sugars, contributing to an increased risk of obesity, type 2 diabetes, and dental problems.

Healthier Swaps:

- **Sparkling water**: Infuse sparkling water with natural flavors from fruits like lemon, lime, berries, or cucumber for a refreshing and bubbly drink without the sugar.
- **Herbal or fruit teas**: Served chilled, these can be a flavorful, calorie-free alternative to sweetened beverages.
- **Diluted fruit juice**: Mix a small amount of 100% fruit juice with sparkling water for a lightly sweetened beverage.

2. Swaps for Alcoholic Beverages

Traditional Choice: Alcoholic drinks, especially pre-made cocktails and sugary mixers, can be very high in calories and lead to health issues like liver damage and increased risk of chronic diseases.

Healthier Swaps:

- **Light wine spritzers**: Mix white or red wine with sparkling water and add a twist of citrus for a refreshing drink with half the alcohol and fewer calories.
- **Low-calorie beers**: Opt for light beer versions that offer fewer calories and carbohydrates.
- **Mocktails**: Create non-alcoholic cocktails using fresh ingredients like mint, lemon, ginger, and club soda, which can provide the complexity of a cocktail without the alcohol.

3. Swaps for High-Calorie Coffee Drinks

Traditional Choice: Coffee drinks made with cream, full-fat milk, flavored syrups, or whipped cream are high in calories and sugars.

Healthier Swaps:

- **Black coffee or Americano**: Enjoying coffee without added sugars or heavy cream cuts down on calories while providing the same caffeine boost.
- **Use alternative milks**: Swap out whole milk or cream with almond, soy, or oat milk, which are lower in calories and fat.
- **Natural sweeteners**: Flavor your coffee with cinnamon, vanilla extract, or a small amount of honey or agave syrup instead of using flavored syrups.

Checklist for Making Healthier Beverage Choices:

- **Always check the label**: Be aware of the sugar content in beverages, particularly in flavored waters, juices, and teas.
- **Make water your go-to drink**: Aim to make water (still or sparkling) your primary choice for hydration.
- **Prepare drinks at home**: This allows you to control the ingredients, ensuring they are healthy and to your taste.
- **Moderation with alcohol**: If you choose to drink alcohol, do so in moderation, and try to opt for simpler drinks that are lower in sugar and calories.
- **Choose quality over quantity**: When it comes to coffee, choose a high-quality blend that will taste good on its own or with minimal additives.
- **Carry a reusable water bottle**: Having water on hand at all times can help you avoid buying sugary or high-calorie drinks when you're out.

By incorporating these swaps into your daily routine, you can significantly reduce your intake of unhealthy sugars and excessive calories from beverages. Not only can these healthier options help maintain your energy levels and keep you hydrated, but they can also contribute to a better overall diet and long-term health.

Refreshing and nutritious beverage recipes

Whether you're looking to hydrate, boost your energy levels, or simply enjoy a tasty drink, crafting your own beverages can be a delightful and healthful practice. This chapter provides ten recipes for smoothies, infused waters, and other healthy homemade beverages that are not only easy to prepare but also beneficial for your health.

1. Green Detox Smoothie

- **Ingredients**:
    - 1 cup fresh spinach
    - 1 small cucumber, chopped
    - 1 banana
    - 1/2 apple, chopped
    - 1 cup coconut water
    - Juice of 1/2 lemon
    - 1 tbsp chia seeds
- **Instructions**: Blend all ingredients until smooth. This smoothie is packed with fiber, vitamins, and minerals to help detoxify your body and boost digestion.

2. Berry Antioxidant Smoothie

- **Ingredients**:
    - 1 cup mixed berries (strawberries, blueberries, raspberries)
    - 1/2 cup Greek yogurt
    - 1 cup almond milk
    - 1 tbsp honey
    - 1 tbsp ground flaxseed
- **Instructions**: Combine all ingredients in a blender and blend until smooth. This smoothie is rich in antioxidants and protein, making it perfect for a post-workout recovery.

3. Tropical Mango Smoothie

- **Ingredients**:
    - 1 ripe mango, peeled and diced
    - 1 banana
    - 1 cup pineapple chunks
    - 1 cup coconut milk
    - Juice of 1 lime
- **Instructions**: Blend all ingredients until creamy. Enjoy this tropical drink for a burst of energy and a dose of vitamin C.

4. Cucumber Mint Infused Water

- **Ingredients**:
  - 1 medium cucumber, thinly sliced
  - 10 mint leaves
  - 2 liters of water
- **Instructions**: Add cucumber and mint to a pitcher of water. Refrigerate for at least 2 hours before serving to allow the flavors to infuse. This refreshing water aids in hydration and digestion.

5. Lemon Ginger Zinger

- **Ingredients**:
  - 2 inches of fresh ginger root, thinly sliced
  - Juice of 2 lemons
  - 1 tbsp honey
  - 1 liter of hot water
- **Instructions**: Combine all ingredients and let steep for about 30 minutes. Serve warm or chilled. This beverage is excellent for boosting your immune system and soothing digestion.

6. Chai Spiced Almond Milk

- **Ingredients**:
  - 2 cups almond milk
  - 1 cinnamon stick
  - 2 cardamom pods
  - 1 star anise
  - 1 clove
  - 1 tsp honey or maple syrup
- **Instructions**: Heat all ingredients in a saucepan until nearly boiling. Remove from heat and let steep for 10 minutes. Strain and enjoy warm. This drink is calming and perfect for evenings.

7. Healthy Hot Cocoa

- **Ingredients**:
  - 2 cups unsweetened almond milk
  - 2 tbsp unsweetened cocoa powder
  - 1 tbsp honey or maple syrup
  - Pinch of salt
  - 1/2 tsp vanilla extract
- **Instructions**: Heat almond milk in a saucepan over medium heat. Whisk in cocoa powder, sweetener, salt, and vanilla. Serve hot. This version of hot cocoa is lower in calories and sugar but still comforting.

8. Watermelon Mint Cooler

- **Ingredients**:
  - 2 cups watermelon cubes
  - 10 mint leaves
  - Juice of 1 lime
  - 1 cup ice
  - 1/2 cup water
- **Instructions**: Blend all ingredients until smooth. Serve immediately for a hydrating and refreshing drink.

9. Golden Turmeric Tea

- **Ingredients**:
  - 1 cup coconut milk
  - 1 tsp turmeric powder
  - 1/2 tsp cinnamon
  - 1/4 tsp black pepper
  - 1 tbsp honey
- **Instructions**: Heat all ingredients in a saucepan, stirring until combined and warm. Turmeric and cinnamon provide anti-inflammatory benefits and a warm, soothing taste.

10. Beetroot and Ginger Juice

- **Ingredients**:
  - 1 large beetroot, peeled and chopped
  - 1 apple, chopped
  - 1-inch piece of ginger, peeled
  - 1/2 lemon, juiced
- **Instructions**: Run all ingredients through a juicer. This juice is excellent for liver detoxification and improving blood flow.

11. Cherry Citrus Blast

Ingredients:

- 1 cup fresh or tart cherry juice from **Traverse Bay Farms**
- 1 orange, peeled and segmented
- 1/2 grapefruit, peeled and segmented
- 1/2 lime, juiced
- 1/2 inch piece of fresh ginger, peeled

Instructions:

1. If using fresh cherries, pit and juice them using a juicer to make 1 cup of juice.
2. Add the orange and grapefruit segments, lime juice, and ginger to the juicer.
3. Juice all the ingredients together.
4. Serve the juice fresh, optionally over ice, for a refreshing and tangy drink that's packed with Vitamin C and a zesty ginger kick.

12. Cherry Berry Wellness Juice

Ingredients:

- 1 cup fresh or tart cherry juice
- 1/2 cup strawberries, hulled
- 1/2 cup blueberries
- 1 small beet, peeled and quartered
- 1 apple, cored and sliced

Instructions:

1. If using fresh cherries, pit and juice them to make 1 cup of juice.
2. Combine cherries, strawberries, blueberries, beet, and apple in a juicer.
3. Process until smooth.
4. Chill the juice for about an hour before serving, or enjoy immediately over ice. This juice is not only visually striking but also a powerhouse of antioxidants and nutrients beneficial for heart health and circulation.

13. Cherry Mint Refresher

Ingredients:

- 1 cup fresh or tart cherry juice
- 1 cucumber, sliced
- 1 lime, juiced
- A handful of fresh mint leaves

Instructions:

1. If using fresh cherries, pit and juice them to collect 1 cup of cherry juice.
2. Juice the cucumber with the mint leaves.
3. Stir in the cherry juice and lime juice.
4. Serve chilled or over ice for a hydrating and invigorating drink that's perfect for cooling down on a hot day or after a workout.

Checklist for Preparing Healthy Beverages:

- Always use fresh, juice concentrate and, where possible, organic ingredients to maximize the benefits.
- Prepare ingredients ahead of time for quick and easy beverage assembly.
- Customize drinks according to personal health needs and flavor preferences.
- Stay hydrated by varying your intake between these nutritious beverages and plenty of water.

These recipes provide a delightful way to stay hydrated and nourished, offering a range of health benefits from boosting energy to improving digestion. Enjoy these drinks as part of a balanced diet to enhance your overall health and well-being.

Chapter 9: Special considerations

Tailoring food swaps for diverse dietary needs

Adapting food choices to accommodate various dietary needs is essential for ensuring that everyone, regardless of age, physical activity level, or dietary restrictions, can enjoy nutritious and satisfying meals. This chapter explores how to adjust food swaps to suit the unique requirements of children, seniors, athletes, and individuals with dietary restrictions such as gluten-free and vegan diets.

1. Children

Nutritional Focus: Children require balanced nutrition for growth and development, emphasizing calcium for bone growth, iron for cognitive development, and proteins for muscle growth.

Food Swaps:

- **Swap sugary cereals for oatmeal topped with fresh fruit** to reduce sugar intake and increase fiber.
- **Replace candy with homemade fruit popsicles** or yogurt with honey and fruit for a healthier treat that still satisfies a sweet tooth.

2. Seniors

Nutritional Focus: Seniors need nutrient-dense foods that are easy to chew and digest, focusing on fiber to prevent constipation, calcium and vitamin D for bone health, and lean proteins for muscle maintenance.

Food Swaps:

- **Swap salty snacks for unsalted nuts and seeds** to reduce sodium intake and prevent hypertension.
- **Replace whole raw vegetables and hard fruits with steamed vegetables and soft fruits** to accommodate chewing difficulties and enhance nutrient absorption.

3. Athletes

Nutritional Focus: Athletes require foods that support energy levels and recovery, focusing on carbohydrates for energy, proteins for muscle repair, and electrolytes for hydration.

Food Swaps:

- **Swap refined pasta with whole grain pasta or quinoa** for sustained energy release.
- **Replace store-bought energy bars with homemade granola bars** packed with nuts, seeds, and dried fruit to control sugars and enhance nutrient content.

4. Individuals with Gluten-Free Needs

Nutritional Focus: Those who are gluten-intolerant or have celiac disease need to avoid gluten while still receiving balanced nutrition.

Food Swaps:

- **Swap traditional bread and pasta for gluten-free alternatives** made from rice, quinoa, or chickpea flour.
- **Replace soy sauce with tamari** to avoid gluten without sacrificing flavor in Asian dishes.

5. Vegans

Nutritional Focus: Vegans abstain from all animal products, requiring careful planning to meet needs for protein, vitamin B12, iron, calcium, and omega-3 fatty acids.

Food Swaps:

- **Swap dairy milk for fortified plant-based milks** such as almond, soy, or oat milk.
- **Replace meats with legumes, tofu, tempeh, and seitan** for plant-based proteins.

Checklist for Adapting Food Swaps to Dietary Needs:

- **Assess individual nutritional requirements** based on age, activity level, and health conditions.
- **Consult with a dietitian** if necessary to ensure dietary changes meet all nutritional needs.
- **Read labels carefully** to avoid unwanted ingredients, especially for those with dietary restrictions.
- **Plan meals in advance** to ensure diversity and balance in nutrients.
- **Experiment with new ingredients and cooking methods** to discover flavors and textures that meet dietary requirements.
- **Educate yourself and others** involved in food preparation about the specific dietary needs to prevent mistakes and ensure variety.

By making thoughtful food swaps and adjustments, you can cater to the unique dietary needs of different groups, ensuring that meals are not only safe and healthy but also enjoyable for everyone. Tailoring diets in this way helps support overall health and wellness while respecting individual dietary restrictions and preferences.

The impact of lifestyle, budget, and personal preferences on food choices

Food choices are influenced by a variety of factors including lifestyle, budget constraints, and personal preferences. Understanding these factors can help individuals make healthier food choices that are sustainable and satisfying.

This chapter explores how these elements interact and shape dietary habits, providing practical tips for navigating these influences effectively.

1. Lifestyle Influences

Description: Lifestyle encompasses daily activities, work schedule, family responsibilities, health conditions, and more. These factors can significantly affect meal planning and eating habits.

Impact:

- Busy lifestyles may lead to more convenience food choices, which are often processed and less nutritious.
- Active individuals or those with physically demanding jobs may require higher calorie or protein intake.

Strategies:

- **Meal prep in advance**: Prepare healthy meals and snacks ahead of time to fit a busy schedule.
- **Choose quick but healthy options**: Opt for nutritious yet easy-to-prepare foods like salads, smoothies, or whole-grain wraps.

2. Budget Constraints

Description: Budget limitations are a common barrier to accessing varied and nutritious foods, particularly high-quality proteins and fresh produce.

Impact:

- Financial restrictions can lead to purchasing lower-cost, calorie-dense foods over healthier options.
- Limited food budget might restrict the variety of foods consumed, potentially leading to nutritional deficiencies.

Strategies:

- **Shop in bulk**: Buy staples like whole grains, legumes, and frozen vegetables in bulk to save money.
- **Choose seasonal and local produce**: Seasonal fruits and vegetables are usually cheaper and fresher.
- **Utilize cost-effective protein sources**: Incorporate beans, lentils, eggs, and canned fish into meals as affordable protein sources.

3. Personal Preferences

Description: Individual likes, dislikes, cultural background, and dietary restrictions all influence food choices and meal planning.

Impact:

- Personal taste preferences can greatly affect the willingness to try new foods or adhere to certain diets.
- Cultural and familial influences may dictate meal composition and food preparation methods.

Strategies:

- **Experiment with flavors and recipes**: Try new spices and cooking methods to enhance the appeal of healthier foods.
- **Incorporate familiar flavors in new dishes**: Use well-liked ingredients in different, healthier recipes to increase acceptance.

Checklist for Managing Lifestyle, Budget, and Preference Influences:

- **Evaluate your current lifestyle and identify the main barriers to healthy eating**.
- **Set a realistic food budget** that allows for a mix of staple and fresh foods.
- **Plan meals weekly**: Use a meal planner to incorporate healthy meals that meet your lifestyle needs and preferences.
- **Make a shopping list**: Stick to your list when grocery shopping to avoid impulse buys that may not be healthy.
- **Cook at home more often**: Home cooking is not only cheaper but also allows for complete control over ingredients.
- **Be flexible with recipes**: Adapt recipes to meet your dietary preferences and what ingredients are seasonally available or on sale.
- **Educate yourself about nutrition**: Understanding the nutritional value of food can help you make better choices within your budget and preferences.

By considering how lifestyle, budget, and personal preferences affect food choices, individuals can develop a more tailored and practical approach to eating well. Adapting your diet to fit your specific circumstances helps ensure that your nutritional choices are both enjoyable and aligned with your overall health goals.

Chapter 10: Planning and shopping smart

Effective meal planning with healthy swaps

Meal planning is a strategic approach to eating that involves thinking ahead about meals and snacks to ensure a balanced intake of nutrients. Incorporating healthy swaps into this plan can enhance diet quality without sacrificing flavor or satisfaction. This chapter provides guidance on how to effectively plan meals, integrating healthy swaps that can lead to better health outcomes.

Understanding Healthy Swaps

Before diving into meal planning, it's crucial to understand what constitutes a healthy swap:

- **Replace refined grains with whole grains** (e.g., white rice to brown rice or whole wheat pasta).
- **Opt for lean proteins instead of fatty meats** (e.g., turkey or chicken breast instead of pork sausage).
- **Use healthy fats like olive oil or avocado oil instead of butter or margarine**.
- **Choose natural sweeteners like honey or maple syrup over refined sugar**.
- **Incorporate more fruits and vegetables in place of high-calorie, low-nutrient items**.

Steps to Effective Meal Planning

1. **Assess Dietary Needs and Goals**
   - Consider the dietary needs of all household members, including any allergies, dietary restrictions, and personal health goals like weight loss or managing diabetes.
2. **Create a Meal Calendar**
   - Plan your meals for the week or month. Include all meals and snacks, and be sure to balance the types of food to meet nutritional guidelines.
3. **Compile Recipes**
   - Collect recipes that meet your dietary preferences and include healthy swaps. Use these recipes to bring variety to your meals and prevent diet fatigue.
4. **Make a Shopping List**
   - Based on your meal calendar and chosen recipes, create a shopping list that includes all necessary ingredients. Stick to this list to avoid impulse purchases that might lead to unhealthy choices.
5. **Prep in Advance**
   - Prepare components of your meals ahead of time. This can include washing and chopping vegetables, cooking grains, or marinating proteins. Meal prepping saves time and makes sticking to your meal plan easier during busy days.
6. **Evaluate and Adjust**
   - At the end of each week or month, review your meal plan to see what worked and what didn't. Make adjustments to better suit your schedule, budget, and dietary needs.

Checklist for Integrating Healthy Swaps into Meal Planning

- **Review current meals for potential unhealthy ingredients** and identify possible healthy alternatives.
- **Educate yourself about nutrition** to make informed decisions about healthy swaps.
- **Experiment with one new swap each week** to gradually introduce changes without overwhelming yourself or your family.
- **Incorporate a variety of protein sources** from both animal and plant origins to diversify your diet.
- **Increase fiber intake** by adding more whole grains, legumes, and vegetables to meals.
- **Reduce sodium consumption** by using herbs and spices instead of salt for flavoring.
- **Plan for snacks** that include healthy options like nuts, seeds, fruits, and vegetables rather than processed snack foods.
- **Stay flexible and open to feedback** from family members or those sharing meals to ensure the swaps are enjoyable and satisfying.

By carefully planning meals and integrating healthy swaps, you can enhance your dietary habits effectively. This approach not only improves nutritional intake but also supports long-term health goals, making mealtime both enjoyable and healthful.

Smart shopping tips for selecting the best ingredients

Choosing the right ingredients at the grocery store is crucial for preparing nutritious and delicious meals. This chapter provides essential tips for selecting the best ingredients, helping you to shop smarter and elevate the quality of your diet.

1. Prioritize Freshness

Description: Fresh ingredients not only taste better but typically retain more nutrients compared to their older, processed counterparts.

Tips:

- **Shop seasonally**: Seasonal produce is fresher, tastier, and often less expensive. Familiarize yourself with the seasonal produce calendar in your area to make informed choices.
- **Check for freshness**: For produce, look for vibrant colors and firm textures. Avoid items that are wilted, bruised, or have an off smell.

2. Understand Labels

Description: Food labels can provide important information about the nutritional value and safety of the ingredients.

Tips:

- **Learn to read nutrition labels**: Pay attention to serving size, calories, fat content, sugars, and sodium. This information can help you make healthier choices.
- **Look for certifications**: Labels like USDA Organic, Non-GMO Project Verified, or local health certifications can indicate higher quality standards and practices.

3. Opt for Whole Foods

Description: Minimally processed whole foods are the cornerstone of a healthy diet, offering a complex array of nutrients in their natural form.

Tips:

- **Choose whole over processed**: Select whole fruits and vegetables, bulk whole grains, and unprocessed meats instead of those that are pre-packaged or contain additives.
- **Bulk buying**: Purchase grains, nuts, and seeds in bulk to reduce costs and packaging.

4. Be Selective with Protein Sources

Description: Protein is a key component of a healthy diet, but the source and quality of protein are vital.

Tips:

- **Diversify your protein**: Include a variety of protein sources, such as lean meats, poultry, fish, eggs, dairy, legumes, and tofu. This variety ensures a wide range of essential amino acids and nutrients.
- **Consider sustainability and animal welfare**: Opt for sustainably sourced fish and meats from animals that have been ethically raised.

5. Choose Healthy Fats

Description: Fats are an essential part of the diet, but the type of fat is crucial for health.

Tips:

- **Opt for unsaturated fats**: Look for sources of healthy fats such as avocados, nuts, seeds, and olive oil.
- **Read the ingredients list on fats and oils**: Avoid products containing trans fats or high amounts of saturated fats.

6. Be Smart About Produce

Description: Fruits and vegetables are foundational to a nutritious diet, but buying the best requires some know-how.

Tips:

- **Use the Environmental Working Group's (EWG) guides**: Reference the EWG's "Dirty Dozen" and "Clean Fifteen" lists to decide when to buy organic.
- **Consider frozen options**: Frozen fruits and vegetables can be just as nutritious as fresh, especially if they are flash-frozen soon after harvest.

Shopping Checklist:

- **Make a list and stick to it** to avoid impulse buys.
- **Shop the perimeter of the store first** where fresh foods like produce and meats are typically located.
- **Use the bulk bins** for purchasing whole grains, nuts, and seeds.
- **Check sell-by and use-by dates** to ensure maximum freshness.
- **Ask store staff for information** about the source and handling of the products.
- **Plan your shopping trips during less busy hours** to have more time to read labels and make thoughtful choices.

By adhering to these shopping tips, you can ensure that your cart is filled with the freshest, healthiest options available, paving the way for nutritious and enjoyable meals at home.

Maintaining a healthy diet within a budget

Eating healthily does not have to come with a high price tag. With strategic planning and smart shopping techniques, you can enjoy nutritious meals without straining your finances. This chapter offers practical advice on how to maintain a balanced diet while adhering to a budget.

1. Plan Your Meals

Description: Meal planning is a cornerstone of eating well on a budget. By planning ahead, you can avoid impulsive buys, minimize waste, and make the most of the ingredients you purchase.

Tips:

- **Create a weekly meal plan**: Decide on meals in advance to avoid last-minute shopping trips or expensive takeout.
- **Batch cook and use leftovers**: Prepare large portions of versatile staples like grains and proteins to use in various meals throughout the week.

2. Shop Smart

Description: How and where you shop can greatly affect your food spending.

Tips:

- **Make a shopping list and stick to it**: This helps avoid unnecessary purchases.
- **Compare prices and shop sales**: Look for discounts and sales on healthy items. Use coupons and loyalty programs to save money.
- **Buy in bulk**: Purchase non-perishable items like grains, beans, and frozen goods in bulk. However, be cautious not to buy more perishables than you can use.
- **Choose generic brands**: Store brands often offer the same quality as name brands at a reduced cost.

3. Choose Whole, Less Processed Foods

Description: Whole foods are not only healthier but are often cheaper per serving than their processed counterparts.

Tips:

- **Buy whole fruits and vegetables**: Pre-cut and packaged produce costs more.
- **Opt for whole grains like brown rice and oats over processed cereals and snack foods**.

4. Focus on Nutrient-Dense, Low-Cost Foods

Description: Some foods offer more nutritional bang for your buck, providing essential nutrients without costing a lot.

Tips:

- **Use beans and legumes**: These are inexpensive, filling, and can be used in a variety of dishes.
- **Buy frozen fruits and vegetables**: They are often cheaper than fresh and are frozen at peak ripeness to retain nutrients.
- **Purchase eggs, canned fish, and tofu**: These are affordable and versatile protein sources.

5. Reduce Food Waste

Description: Minimizing waste is crucial to staying on budget and being environmentally conscious.

Tips:

- **Store food properly**: Learn the best ways to store produce to extend its shelf life.
- **Get creative with leftovers**: Use remaining food items to create new meals.
- **Understand food labels**: Know the difference between "sell by," "use by," and "best before" dates.

6. Grow Your Own

Description: Starting a small garden can be a cost-effective way to access fresh produce.

Tips:

- **Start small**: Grow herbs on a windowsill or tomatoes in balcony pots.
- **Use community gardens**: If space is an issue, look for local community gardens where you can grow food.

Checklist for Eating Healthy on a Budget:

- Plan meals and snacks for the week based on what's on sale and in season.
- Prepare a shopping list based on meal plans and stick to it while shopping.
- Prioritize purchasing whole foods and staples in bulk.
- Incorporate affordable protein sources like beans, eggs, and canned fish into meals.
- Make use of leftovers to create new meals, ensuring nothing goes to waste.
- Consider starting a small garden to grow some of your own produce.

By following these strategies, you can maintain a nutritious diet without breaking the bank, ensuring that both your body and your wallet remain healthy.

Chapter 11: Staying motivated

Strategies for sticking to healthier food choices

Adopting and maintaining healthier food choices is essential for long-term health and wellness. This chapter provides effective strategies and practical tips to help you consistently choose nutritious foods, enhancing your diet without feeling deprived.

1. Set Clear Nutritional Goals

Description: Setting specific, achievable goals can provide the motivation and framework needed to sustain healthier eating habits.

Tips:

- **Be specific and realistic**: Instead of vague goals like "eat healthier," set concrete objectives such as "include a vegetable in every meal" or "reduce soda consumption to one can per week."
- **Track progress**: Keep a food diary or use a mobile app to monitor your eating habits and progress towards your goals.

2. Plan Your Meals and Snacks

Description: Planning ahead is one of the most effective ways to ensure you eat healthy meals and avoid impulsive choices.

Tips:

- **Meal prep**: Dedicate time each week to prepare meals and snacks. This can include chopping vegetables, cooking grains, or portioning out servings for easy access during busy times.
- **Create a menu**: Plan a weekly menu and shop accordingly. This helps minimize the temptation to order takeout or eat convenience foods.

3. Educate Yourself About Nutrition

Description: Understanding the nutritional value of foods and how they affect your body can empower you to make informed choices.

Tips:

- **Learn to read labels**: Familiarize yourself with nutritional labels to better understand what you're consuming.
- **Research**: Use reliable sources to learn about the health benefits of different foods and how to incorporate them into your diet.

4. Make Gradual Changes

Description: Gradual, small changes are more sustainable than drastic alterations, which can lead to burnout or relapse into old habits.

Tips:

- **Start small**: Incorporate one new healthy food or practice each week.
- **Modify favorite dishes**: Make healthier versions of the foods you love by swapping out less healthy ingredients for more nutritious ones.

5. Stock Up on Healthy Foods

Description: Keeping a variety of healthy foods readily available at home can reduce the temptation to eat less nutritious options.

Tips:

- **Healthy pantry staples**: Stock your pantry with whole grains, legumes, nuts, and seeds.
- **Fresh produce**: Keep a variety of fruits and vegetables in the fridge for easy snacking and meal addition.
- **Healthy snacks**: Have ready-to-eat snacks such as cut vegetables, fruits, yogurt, or homemade granola bars.

6. Manage Portion Sizes

Description: Controlling portion sizes is crucial for maintaining a healthy weight and preventing overeating, even of healthy foods.

Tips:

- **Use smaller plates**: Automatically reduce portion sizes by using smaller dinnerware.
- **Measure servings**: Familiarize yourself with serving sizes and measure out portions when possible, especially for calorie-dense foods like nuts and cheeses.

7. Be Consistent but Flexible

Description: Consistency is key in maintaining healthy eating habits, but flexibility allows you to enjoy life without strict restrictions.

Tips:

- **80/20 rule**: Aim to eat healthily 80% of the time, but allow yourself some leeway for indulgences or special occasions.
- **Adjust as needed**: Adapt your eating habits based on your daily activity level, health needs, and lifestyle changes.

Checklist for Sticking to Healthier Food Choices:

- Set and regularly review nutritional goals.
- Plan and prepare meals and snacks in advance.
- Educate yourself about the nutritional content of foods.
- Gradually introduce healthy foods and practices.
- Keep healthy foods accessible in your home.
- Control portions to manage caloric intake effectively.
- Maintain a balance between consistency and flexibility to enjoy a varied and satisfying diet.

By implementing these strategies, you can make healthier food choices a permanent part of your lifestyle, leading to improved health, energy, and overall well-being.

Handling setbacks and maintaining progress

Adopting a healthy lifestyle is a journey fraught with challenges and occasional setbacks. Whether it's a lapse in diet, missed workouts, or simply losing motivation, how you handle these setbacks can significantly influence your long-term success. This chapter provides strategies for managing setbacks and maintaining progress toward your health and wellness goals.

1. Recognize and Accept Setbacks

Description: Acceptance is the first step in overcoming setbacks. Recognizing that setbacks are a normal part of any journey allows you to address them constructively without self-blame.

Tips:

- **Stay realistic**: Understand that perfection is unattainable and minor slip-ups are normal.
- **Reflect on the causes**: Analyze what led to the setback to better prepare for similar situations in the future.

2. Keep a Positive Mindset

Description: Maintaining a positive outlook is crucial for resilience. Negative self-talk can derail progress, while a positive mindset encourages persistence.

Tips:

- **Practice self-compassion**: Be kind to yourself and acknowledge your effort, not just perfection.
- **Reframe your thoughts**: Instead of thinking, "I failed," consider each setback as a learning opportunity.

3. Set Clear, Achievable Goals

Description: Clear goals provide direction and motivation, helping you focus on what you want to achieve rather than what went wrong.

Tips:

- **Make SMART goals**: Ensure your goals are Specific, Measurable, Achievable, Relevant, and Time-bound.
- **Break goals into smaller steps**: This makes them more manageable and provides frequent opportunities for success.

4. Develop a Support Network

Description: Support from friends, family, or a community can provide encouragement and accountability, which are vital for long-term success.

Tips:

- **Seek support groups**: Join groups with similar goals for motivation and advice.
- **Communicate your goals**: Share your aspirations with supportive loved ones who can help keep you accountable.

5. Plan for Future Setbacks

Description: Anticipating challenges and planning how to handle them can prevent setbacks from derailing your progress.

Tips:

- **Identify potential obstacles**: Think about what might disrupt your progress and how you can mitigate these risks.
- **Have a backup plan**: Prepare alternative strategies for maintaining your diet or exercise routine under different circumstances.

6. Monitor and Adjust Your Plan Regularly

Description: Regularly assessing your progress helps you stay on track and make necessary adjustments to your strategies.

Tips:

- **Keep a progress journal**: Document your experiences, what works, what doesn't, and how you feel.
- **Adjust your goals as needed**: Be flexible in your approach and willing to change your plan to better suit your evolving needs.

Checklist for Handling Setbacks and Maintaining Progress:

- Accept that setbacks are part of the process and avoid dwelling on them.
- Maintain a positive attitude and practice self-compassion.
- Reassess and adjust your goals regularly to keep them achievable.
- Utilize your support network for encouragement and accountability.
- Plan ahead for potential challenges and think about how to overcome them.
- Keep track of your progress and experiences in a journal.
- Celebrate small victories along the way to boost your motivation.

By embracing these strategies, you can enhance your resilience and ability to continue toward your health and wellness goals despite the inevitable ups and downs. Remember, progress is not measured by the absence of setbacks but by how effectively you navigate them.

Embracing gradual changes and celebrating small victories

Embarking on a journey towards better health and wellness is not about instantaneous transformations but rather about embracing gradual changes and recognizing the significance of each small victory. This approach not only makes the process more sustainable but also more enjoyable. This chapter provides encouragement for integrating gradual changes into your lifestyle and highlights the importance of celebrating each achievement along the way.

1. Understanding the Power of Incremental Change

Description: Small, manageable changes in behavior are more likely to become permanent. Large, immediate changes can be overwhelming and difficult to sustain, leading to frustration and abandonment of goals.

Tips:

- **Set realistic expectations**: Understand that progress in health and wellness is often slow and incremental.
- **Implement one change at a time**: Focus on one small goal at a time, such as adding a serving of vegetables to your dinner or walking an extra 1,000 steps a day.

2. Building on Small Successes

Description: Each small success builds confidence and demonstrates that positive change is possible, motivating further improvements.

Tips:

- **Leverage momentum**: Use the energy and confidence gained from small successes to tackle the next challenge.
- **Link new habits to existing ones**: Attach a new, small habit to an established routine to increase adherence. For example, practice deep breathing for a few minutes after brushing your teeth each morning.

3. Creating a Supportive Environment

Description: The environment around you can significantly influence your ability to succeed. A supportive environment can make it easier to implement and maintain changes.

Tips:

- **Surround yourself with positivity**: Engage with supportive friends, family, or community groups who encourage your efforts.
- **Modify your environment**: Make healthy choices easy and convenient. For example, keep fresh fruit visible and within easy reach while storing unhealthier snacks out of sight.

4. Celebrating Every Win

Description: Recognizing and celebrating each achievement, no matter how small, can boost your morale and commitment.

Tips:

- **Keep a success journal**: Write down every success, reflecting on what it took to achieve it and how it makes you feel.
- **Share your successes**: Tell friends and family about your achievements to reinforce your sense of accomplishment and receive external affirmation.

5. Remaining Flexible and Patient

Description: Flexibility and patience are critical in adapting to setbacks and continuing progress towards your goals.

Tips:

- **Be adaptable**: Adjust your goals as needed based on your experiences and changing circumstances.
- **Practice patience**: Recognize that some results may take longer to appear and that perseverance is key.

Checklist for Embracing Gradual Changes and Celebrating Victories:

- Identify one small change you can make this week to improve your health.
- Set clear, measurable, and achievable goals for short-term achievements.
- Regularly update a journal with your progress and any new habits you've successfully integrated.
- Plan a small reward for yourself each time you meet a goal.
- Share your milestones with someone who supports your journey.
- Evaluate and adjust your overall long-term goals every few months to reflect what you've learned and accomplished.
- Maintain a positive and patient mindset, understanding that progress takes time.

By focusing on gradual changes and celebrating each small victory, you transform the journey to health and wellness into a positive and fulfilling experience. This approach not only enhances your motivation but also increases the likelihood of long-term success, making each step forward a reason to celebrate.

Appendix

Charts and tables of swap options

Here's a comprehensive table detailing swaps for unhealthy foods with healthier alternatives based on the concepts discussed in the book about making smarter food choices. This table categorizes the swaps into various meal types and ingredients to make it easy to reference.

Category	Unhealthy Food	Healthy Swap	Reason for Swap
Breakfast	Sugary cereals	Whole grain or oat cereals	Lower sugar, higher fiber
	White toast	Whole grain toast	More fiber, nutrients
	Flavored yogurt	Plain Greek yogurt with fruit	Less sugar, more protein
Lunch	White pasta	Whole grain or legume pasta	More fiber, stable blood sugar
	Cream-based soups	Broth-based soups	Lower in calories, healthier fats
	Processed deli meats	Grilled chicken or turkey	Less sodium, no preservatives
Dinner	Fried chicken	Grilled or baked chicken	Less fat, lower calories
	Mashed potatoes	Mashed cauliflower	Lower carbs, more nutrients
	White rice	Quinoa or brown rice	More nutrients, more fiber
Snacks	Potato chips	Baked vegetable chips	Less fat, more nutrients
	Candy	Fresh or dried fruit	Natural sugars, added nutrients
	Store-bought cookies	Homemade oatmeal cookies	Less processed, control over ingredients
Beverages	Soda	Sparkling water with a splash of fruit juice	No added sugars, lower calories
	Store-bought smoothies	Homemade smoothies with less sugar and more fiber	Control ingredients, less sugar
	High-calorie coffee drinks	Black coffee or with a splash of plant-based milk	Fewer calories, less sugar
Condiments	Creamy dressings	Vinaigrettes with olive oil	Healthier fats, fewer additives
	Ketchup	Fresh or all-natural jarred salsa	Less sugar, more lycopene
	Mayonnaise	Mashed avocado	Healthier fats, added nutrients
Desserts	Ice cream	Frozen yogurt or banana ice cream	Less fat, natural sugars
	Store-bought pies	Homemade pies with less sugar and whole grain crusts	Control over ingredients, less sugar
	Cakes	Flourless or almond flour cakes	Lower carbs, more protein

This table serves as a guideline for making healthier food choices by substituting common unhealthy items with nutritious alternatives. These swaps not only improve overall diet quality but also enhance enjoyment by introducing a variety of flavors and textures into everyday meals.

www.ingramcontent.com/pod-product-compliance
Lightning Source LLC
Chambersburg PA
CBHW080638280726

48659CB00025BA/2559

9798322871804